M360

CLINICAL FITNESS

M360

CLINICAL FITNESS
Metabolic Fitness for Life

TIM BARNES

To order additional copies of this book, contact:
Xlibris
1-888-795-4274
www.Xlibris.com
Orders@Xlibris.com
782629

CONTENTS

FOREWORD

What is the common denominator we all share on this earth as humans?

How many hours are there in a day? We all share a 24 hour day don't we?

What is the most important part of our day, your day? _____

Think... What is the MOST important part of our DAY?

How many of you said sleep? By far the most important part of our day as humans is sleep! We must recover, recharge and renew or we will implode and along the way lose our health at every level you analyze it.

This book is about that day, your day, and what you do with the remaining 16 hours after you master your sleep. Mastering your lifestyle starts with quality sleep in the range of 8 hours per 24 hours. Metabolic health is the point of this book.

- Metabolic Health starts with Sleep, Recovery and Renewal
- Metabolic Health starts with quality production of Energy and Healthy Mitochondria to produce sustainable energy.
- The energy currency of our human bodies is ATP.
- How well do you produce it and support the metabolic system that creates it, that creates and supports LIFE?

ATP is a complex organic chemical that participates in many processes. Found in all forms of life, ATP is often referred to as the **"Molecular unit of Currency"** of intracellular energy transfer. There is **NOT** a genius on earth that would disagree to Sleep Recovery and Energy Production being the cornerstones of optimal health and human performance.

As of this writing here at 4:43 am on a Monday, I am fresh back from spending the weekend at the **United States Olympic Training Center** in Colorado Springs. I was honored to assist as a Performance Facilitator to pick the **Next Olympic Hopeful. #nextolympichopeful**

The **US Olympic Committee** put this program together that will air on **NBCsn** and **NBC** annually. As evaluators we were faced with 90 finalists of men and women ages 18-30 who were selected from various programs around the country for a 3 day assessment of their skills and Olympic abilities. This experience is what is fueling my writing of this forward or preface to this book.

90 Olympic Hopefuls all in one place seeking just a few elite spots of opportunity. I asked several coaches and athletes the same question I am asking YOU.

What is most important part of your day? Each and everyone I asked looked for some fancy answer that would impress me and they missed the mark of **SLEEP.** I asked the same people what the single most important element of their waking pursuit of high performance was and I got the same non-specific drifting answers. The single most important element of waking pursuit of higher performance is **ENERGY** and your ability to produce **ATP.** Without this ability you are like a CAR without GAS. You are DEAD in the WATER.

Sleep and Energy are critical to mastering your lifestyle, so by default what you do in the course of our waking day and HOW We FEED the NEED of what it is that we do is CRITICAL. Are we optimizing our selection of food? Are you choosing foods with high Nutraceutical Value? Are you taking it upon yourself to better understand Functional Whole Foods and the Value they hold for our health, performance and recovery?

What about Physical Activity and Exercise have we taken time to understand the principles cornerstones of:

- Intensity
- Duration
- Frequency

Are we learning that historically we do 2- things all too well- **Nothing** and **Too Much** and the sad truth that we can be fit for a time being, but also be very unhealthy. Are we spending too much time above and below the very intensities that will improve our Fat Metabolism?

Are we Fat Adapted?

How are we managing stress? Are we taking time to deactivate our Sympathetic Nervous System and activate our Parasympathetic Nervous System to effectively relax and renew daily?

Are we utilizing all the wonderful opportunities to enhance or metabolism by:

- Intermittent Fasting
- Dry Brushing
- Hot Baths
- Yoga and Tai Chi
- Time Restricted eating
- Reference Point Training
- Utilizing the Magic of FFA Training
- Stimulating metabolic rate with ATP Training
- Challenging our Aerobic Capacity with LBP Training

- Lowering our Blood Pressure with key Nutraceuticals like Beets and Beet juice.

This is just a short list of things you can employ into your lifestyle that will reap a cascade of positive metabolic responses that will reduce Stress and Improve Health and Performance as we reduce and eliminate Chronic Inflammation and Oxidation.

With this approach activated we can begin to reduce chronic conditions that lead to Chronic Disease. REMEMBER: Total US Healthcare at last count was $3.2 Trillion Dollars with $2.9 Trillion of that being spent on Chronic Disease that by definition is not curable with Vaccination or Pharmaceuticals. Chronic Disease is a Chronic Condition of POOR LIFESTYLE.

In closing: Why do we skip over the most important elements or components of our Lifestyle in Pursuit of a Goal? Don't **SLEEP** and our systems that produce **ENERGY/LIFE** deserve some attention?

With all the fancy programs of health and performance out there from your corner gym to the hallowed ground of the US Olympic Training center isn't Metabolic Health and Performance really **GROUND ZERO** to our proclivity toward success at everything we do?

In this book and in our podcast's we simply address sound bites of information on various topics for you to explore and potentially adopt into your lifestyle. We call them components of your lifestyle.

What are the components of your 16 hour day?

After sleep, work, and family, what do you have left in terms of time? You very quickly see it is NOT a long complex period of time.

How do you use this time?

What do you choose to assign power in your life? What are your motivations and directions? What do you base your direction on? Are you lost, or are you addressing your lifestyle, exercise, diet and stress management from a position of intelligence?

Learning is the KEY toward making better decisions, making better choices and modifying your behavior to possess the contagious *ESSENCE of SUCCESS*. We simply DO NOT know what we DO NOT KNOW, but we can learn.

You must take it upon yourself to seek, and Master Your Lifestyle to achieve **Metabolic Fitness for Life.**

Use this book as source to prompt your own personal discover, use our resources at:

1. Podcast @ **"Power 2 Learn"** on iTunes and Google Play for our podcasts and interviews with everyday client success stories.
2. Blogs at **www.metafit.life**
3. Email me at **tim@metafit.life** or
4. Join our sessions at our **M360 Fitness Clinic** near you.

SECTION #1

Lifestyle

Components of Optimal Health & Human Performance

LIFESTYLE #1

Components of a Healthy Lifestyle & Metabolism

What is your definition of lifestyle? _____

Definition According to Webster's Dictionary:

"Way of life by a person or group of persons".

Australian physiologist Alfred Alder introduced the term **"Lifestyle"** with the meaning of **"A Persons Basic character as established earlier in childhood"**. Lifestyle is how you set up, and live your life- day by day. Lifestyle is the gestalt of what you choose to pursue- based on your own unique value system of needs, wants and motivations. These components determine our:

- **Culture**
- **Family**
- **Reference group**
- **Social class**

What have we taught ourselves and what are we teaching our kids about a metabolically -healthy lifestyle?

Does your Lifestyle FEEL GOOD? _____

Here is **WHY** we created - Metafit Life 360- short for:

Metabolic Fitness for Life or M360

M360 was inspired to me by the late **Dr. Mark Potzler**, see short television interview with Dr. Potzler at: **www.metafit.life.**

Picture this scenario: Patient goes to healthcare provider and asks the Dr:

How can I improve my health and get off of these medications?

The doctor says: *"Change your lifestyle, diet, and start exercising"*, but what exactly does that mean? People are lost! The very healthcare providers themselves are lost! It is truly a case of the blind leading the blind! What happens next?

Specifically: *"What should I do the patient ask"?*

The problem with this scenario, is the patient population, **does not know what to do**. The healthcare providers do a great job of treating infectious disease and prescribing pharmaceuticals, but not at treating *Chronic Conditions* that lead to *Chronic Disease.* Chronic Conditions that represent the **BULK** of our annual USA Healthcare costs (over $2.9 trillion Dollars of $3.2 trillion total).

To complicate the scenario even farther, the patient may seek fitness with one of the many gym rat infestations scattered around every town that has some overweight, chronically inflamed- muscle head gulping down creatine and barking out **"Push-Push"** as if someone were having a baby. This is just wrong at every level of intelligence! We can do better, we can seek a more intelligent **"Evidence based Process"**, a Systematic

Process that is scientifically based to **TARGET** and **DOCUMENT** specific improvements to a variety of -**Clinical Biomarkers**.

Here are 15 Modalities of your Health and Performance we will define in our book, simplify in our interactive workbook, and track you through in our 8-12 week total immersion program:

1. **Modality #1 Lifestyle: A Sustainable Cornerstone Structure of life**.
   a. Arranging our day for Sustainable Structure/Behavior Modification.
   b. New Healthy Components of each and <u>EVERY</u> single day
      i. Exercise/Physical Activity
      ii. Diet/ Nutrition
      iii. Stress Management Rest, Relaxation and Recovery
   c. Out with the old in with the new: Habits, Addictions & Ignorance.
   d. What is Killing Us as a Species?
      i. Heart Disease
      ii. Cancer (malignant tumor growth)
      iii. Respiratory Disease
   e. Why are we Chronically Diseased and Pre Maturely Aging?
      i. Inflammation
      ii. Oxidation
      iii. Epigenetic Factors and Poor Education.
2. **Modality #2 Physical Activities & Exercise: Finding a Sustainable Structure of Activity/ Exercise.**
   a. Time for Physical Activities and making time to Exercise
   b. Variety and a sense of Purpose by Reference point accountability and wearable tracking technology
   c. Concept of: Intensity, Duration and Frequency
3. **Modality #3 Diet & Nutrition: Finding Sustainable Structure of Nutrition for your NEW Life.**
   a. Feeding Metabolic Need, Nutraceutical over Pharmaceutical.
   b. What & When to Eat and Why by Macro Nutrient

c. Anabolic vs. Catabolic Nutritional needs and States

4. **Modality #4 Inflammation: How to Bio-Hack our Metabolism and lower Chronic Inflammation**
   a. Why are we Chronically Inflamed?
   b. How can we reduce dangerous Chronic Inflammation?

5. **Modality #5 Oxidation: How to Bio-Hack the Process of Aging and Lower Oxidative Stress.**
   a. What is Oxidative Stress, why do we have it?
   b. What we are doing about it?

6. **Modality #6 Metabolic Fundamentals: Energy Producing Systems**
   a. **Glycolic**: Carbohydrate utilizing Metabolic Pathway and 36 ATP Units of Energy.
   b. **Lypolic:** Fat Burning Metabolic Pathway and 108 ATP Units of Energy.

7. **Modality #7 Hormone Balance: Metabolic Managers and Optimum Health.**
   a. Insulin and Glucagon (fat storage & utilization)
   b. Ghrelin and Cortisol (hunger & stress)

8. **Modality #8 Mitochondrial Health: Activating your Energy Powerhouse.**
   a. Exercise and Physical activities affect on Mitochondria
   b. Diet and Nutrition's affect on Mitochondria

9. **Modality #9 Ultimate Biological Energy Efficiency: Adopting a Fat Adapted Metabolism**
   a. Burning Fat for Fuel
   b. A place and time for Sugar Fuel

10. **Modality #10 Intermittent Fasting: Autophagy & Optimal Cellular Efficiency.**
    a. Effects of IM and TMR (Time Restricted Eating)
    b. Process and structure of placement in your week

11. **Modality #11 DNA/Genetics: You have more say in your genetic outcome than you may think!**
    a. Epigenetic definitions
    b. Epigenetic interventions and genetic expression

12. **Modality #12 FFA Training: Logic of Metabolic Building from the Bottom UP**
    a. Fat burning Lifestyle and Time Restricted Eating
    b. Fat Burning FFA Exercise and Physical Activities
13. **Modality #13 Aerobic Capacity: We are "Aerobes" on an Oxygen Planet Earth**
    a. ATP Training and Vitality of Power
    b. Optimum Utilization of Abundant Power and Energy to LIVE!
14. **Modality #14 Sleep Recovery & Stress Mgmt: The Lost Link of Load and Recover Training**.
    a. Heart Rate Variability (HRV) and Sleep Quality
    b. Sleep deprivation, and circadian misalignment-sympathetic overstimulation, hormonal imbalance, and **INFLAMMATION & OXIDATION!**
    c. Yoga and Tai Chi…
15. **Modality #15 Healthspan and the Process of Aging: Fountain of youth or even Immortality?**
    a. Calorie Restriction and Fasting
    b. Hydration-Electrolytes Protein and Fat Adapted Composition and Condition for Life

What is killing us?

Some 75% of all deaths in the United States result from just 10 causes, with 3 of these accounting for over 50% of all deaths. Over a span of the last 5 years, the causes of death in the United States have been fairly consistent.

1. Heart disease - 23.4% of total deaths:

> The leading cause of death for both men and women in the United States is Heart Disease. Heart Disease is also the #1 cause of death worldwide. Just over half of the deaths that occur as a result of heart disease are in men.

2. Cancer - 22.5% of total deaths:

> Cancer is defined as uncontrolled growths and the spread of abnormal cells. If cancer is not controlled, it can interrupt life-sustaining systems and result in death.

The leading causes of death from cancer for <u>males</u> are:

- Lung and bronchus
- Prostate
- Rectal/Colon

Leading causes of death from cancer for <u>females</u>:

- Lung and bronchus
- Breast
- Colon and rectum

Research indicates that 1/3 of cancer cases occur in countries like the U.S. that are economically developed. Studies indicate that cancer is related to being:

- Overweight
- Obese
- Inactive(sedentary)
- With a routine of poor nutrition.

3. Chronic lower respiratory disease -5.6% of total deaths:

Chronic lower respiratory diseases (CLRD) represent a variety of lung conditions that cause blocked or partially block airflow, that result in breathing-related issues. The primary CLRD is chronic obstructive pulmonary disease (COPD).

- **These Conditions are <u>PREVENTABLE</u>!**
- **Why are we so <u>Chronically Diseased?</u>**

According to the highly respected **Cleveland Clinic** most **Chronic Illness** is a product of poor lifestyle choices!

1. **Poor <u>planning</u> of Lifestyle Components**
2. **Lack of <u>proper</u> Physical Activity and Exercise**
3. **Poor Diet/Nutrition and a <u>Lack</u> of Nutraceutical Education.**
4. **Inadequate relief of <u>Chronic Stress</u>**

Don't believe us?

Here is what the <u>Cleveland Clinic</u> says is behind Chronic Disease:

"POOR LIFESTYLE CHOICES"!

Broken Relationship between Doctor and Patient Population

"Even though doctors encourage healthful behaviors to help prevent or manage many chronic medical conditions, many patients are inadequately prepared to either start or maintain these appropriate, healthy changes.

Most patients understand the reasoning behind a healthy lifestyle even if they don't understand the disease processes that can occur when they don't maintain healthy habits.

Despite an understanding of what constitutes a healthy lifestyle, many patients lack the behavioral skills they need to apply everyday to sustain these good habits." Cleveland Clinic

> *"Inadequately prepared to either start or maintain These appropriate, healthy changes"...*

Million Dollar Question: So what are <u>YOU</u> Going To Do About It?

Bingo- Metafit Life 360 (**M360**) is here to help you **PREVENT** and eliminate conditions that lead to chronic disease, by educating and learning as we have **FUN** in a group and:

• **<u>Feel Good</u> About enjoying a Healthier Process of Life!**

What we need is total immersion into a Metabolic Fitness Program. All components must point to sustainable: **Metabolic Fitness for Life!**

M360 is a: *Comprehensive - Group Based -Hands on Intervention Program!*

You need a group of like minded folks to wean yourself **OFF SUGAR**, to **MODIFY YOUR BEHAVIOR** and to **EDUCATE** and arm yourself with the tools you need to **SUSTAIN** new modalities of life. We are here to assist you in your journey- in the following modes:

- **By** book as a reference manual or guide to operate from.
- **By** Total Immersion Workbook. Hands on step by step program of action.
- **By** passive learning and awareness via **FREE** Podcast as you walk and move.
- **By** email communication with me at: tim@metafit.life
- **By** Metafit Life 360 on Face Book.
- **By** website: www.metafit.life Blog
- **By** Seminars, hourly and 8-12-week immersion blocks you can attend.
- **By** hourly Sessions to maintain and sustain performance.

You can do **M360** alone or with as much of our help as you choose to solicit. Make **NO** mistake about it, **change in some cases is literally a matter of LIFE or DEATH**, in some cases a total educational and behavioral rehabilitation is needed.

Total Immersion from time to time is what we all need, to wake up and realize the many things we can do daily, that will direct an ongoing cascade of healthy change!

Look around, what do you see? We as a society are killing ourselves with consumption of sugar and overconsumption in general. This truly is a life or death scenario, in many cases a scenario of **CHOICE** with immediate consequences. Immediate steps to better health, or a future of long-term chronic disease? Are you happy in your skin? How will you look, feel and operate metabolically in 20 years?

Take it upon yourself to learn new, exciting ways to improve your metabolism!

Lifestyle is modality #1 to help you define how you arrange your day, week, month and year. The key is to establish productive sustainable habits and routines- when you go to bed, when you wake up, when you eat, when you work, when you exercise and how to relax and recover? Together this makes for how you spend **168** hours a week.

How do we spend our 168 hr week, our 16 hours day? _____

What is the **STRUCTURE** of our **LIFE?** This is our Lifestyle!

Sample 168 hr week: Sleep 56 hours, Work 56 hours, Family 14 hours, Exercise 14 Hours, Eat 14 hours, and Personal Relaxation 14 hours?

We really only have **16 hours a day** to work with when you take 24 minus 8 for sleeping. **Think about that?** A simple 16 hours a day to design and arrange into a more productive sequence of components that can totally change your health and wellness landscape forever.

What is our daily schematic? _____

As you can see, time is limited and must be utilized wisely. This is our challenge. This is your challenge! The good news is there are only 16 hours to organize. We are habitual by nature, so once you get the 16 correct, they will tend to repeat themselves as days become weeks, and weeks become years! We are much better off already by simple becoming **aware** of how precious and limited time is. We do not have time for frivolous- meaningless diets- exercise or misleading information. Let's get it right, let's learn new ways to get motivated and improve the quality and longevity of our health and life.

Workout programs for the most part <u>DO NOT WORK</u> long term!

Why? _____

12 years of my life I spent as the owner/operator of one of the world's first group fitness studios by the name of *Therafit Personalized Training*. I had hundreds of clients and we were very successful, but one of my biggest frustrations was the fact that I only had the clients 3 or maybe 5 hours a week out of 168 total hours. The good we can do in 3-5 hours is nice, but the damage they could do in the other 163-165 hours was devastating.

M360 can keep you out of the Hospital

I am **ON FIRE** with passion to share what I have learned these past 6 years. Information about physical activity, moderate and measured exercise, stress reduction and sure fired methods of reducing Inflammation and Oxidation. There are so many simple and fun interventions we can execute daily that will optimize our health and keep us **<u>OUT</u>** of the doctor's office, out of the hospital, or even worse, out of the morgue!

Chronic Disease is defined as a condition that cannot be addressed with vaccination or medicine. These are conditions of **<u>POOR</u>** lifestyle management.

What are the Components of your Lifestyle? _____

Lifestyle is the framework of your metaphorical home, and within that home are the other sections of this book. This section will brief on every topic, with remaining sections detailing information on each lifestyle component. This book is meant as a point of reference to our workbooks, and daily programs.

Please, **YOU MUST TAKE IT UPON YOURSELF**- to get involved in your **own** process of health and wellness by raising your **own** bar of education and personal performance as it pertains to 4 simple sections:

- **Lifestyle Structure and Choice**
- **Physical Activity and Exercise**
- **Diet and Nutrition**
- **Mindset-Motivation-Relaxation and Meditation**

Every step of this book is targeted at preventing - eliminating, even reversing Chronic Disease and Optimizing your Health and Human Performance by:

- Reducing Inflammation & Oxidation. (ROS) reactive oxygen species/free radicals.
- Improving your Heart Rate Variability. (HRV)
- Improving your Post Exercise Recovery Rate. (PERR)
- Optimizing & Improving your Lean Mass & Strength to Weight Ratio.(STWR)
- Lowering your % of Fat Mass (FM) improving Lean Mass (LM).
- Improve your ability to utilize stored body fat with the objective to become **Fat Adapted** and **Energy Efficient** through FFA/ATP/LBP-RPT Training.
- Improve your overall ability to **DEACTIVATE** your Sympathetic Autonomic Nervous System (SANS).
- Improve your overall ability to **ACTIVATE** your Parasympathetic Autonomic Nervous System (PANS)\

We all have 168 hours each week of our lives:

We all have 168 hours a week to structure our life. We all have individual goals to achieve. The pedagogy we share is a systematic structure of time and process (lifestyle) that targets the underlying causes of **Chronic Disease** with the common goal of all readers and program participants to:

Optimize Health, Wellness and achieve: Metabolic Fitness for Life.

This is our common **Metabolic Health**, our **Metabolic Life** (Metafit. life). It all starts at the cellular level, as my partner Keith Jackson says: **"One Cell at a Time".**

Metabolic Evolution

Evolutionarily speaking, humankind has metabolically changed less than .02% in the last 40,000 plus years. We are destroying our metabolism and disrespecting the gift of life, that is kept running by our metabolic process.

Our metabolism is struggling to save our lives, as we over feed it with:

- **Too much** sugar
- **Too much** stress
- **Too much** toxic chemical in food and:
- **Too much** food in general, fed too often

We spend little to **NO TIME** in these healthy states:

1. **NO TIME** in an **UNFED** State (Fat Adaption)
2. **NO TIME** in a state of **Autophagy** (Cellular Cleansing)
3. **NO TIME** in a state of **Gluconeogenesis** (Conversion of Fat Glycerol)
4. **NO TIME** in a state of **Beta Oxidation** of our **Fat Storage** (adiposity) into **Human Energy (ATP).**

YOU MAY ASK: "Why are we, as a <u>SOCIETY</u>- SICK and FAT"?

It is crazy that so many people are walking around obese, complaining about lack of energy. Fat is a key energy substrate, and the metabolic process of converting it to ATP energy will reduce body fat, and increase performance at every level of:

- **Power**
- **Vitality**
- **Function**

We can all enjoy better performance at every level of life. The underlining problem with our **Chronically Diseased World** is we are **NO LONGER** fat adapted, so we (General Mass Population) have **NO ACCESS** to the huge store of energy we are lugging around in the form of adipose tissue.

This very adiposity is also further making us Chronically Ill. It is truly a crazy scenario when you take time to understand it. Don't you think it is about time to educate, to learn, and to adopt new behaviors? New behaviors based on simple facts of biology that could bring happiness and change our personal and cumulative wellness landscape? **If not for yourself, or community, what about your children?**

Show me the ENERGY support and care for your Mitochondrial Fitness:

- Do you know how our mitochondria work?
- Do you even know what they are?
- Do you know how essential mitochondrial health is to your:
    - **Personal energy** to accomplish life works
    - **Cognitive Focus** to stay mentally sharp & healthy
    - **Power** to perform athletically, from champion to weekend warrior.
    - **Vitality** to achieve day to day goals and enjoy recreation.
    - **Function** to efficiently achieve- basic daily activities.
    - **Metabolism** in general?

If you only had one car in the course of your life, I think you would be better aware of its operational status, and take better care of it -even baby it- with preventative maintenance, oil changes and proper clean fuels to improve gas mileage and performance over time. **Why don't we do this with our bodies?**

- Who here is getting any **YOUNGER?**
- Who here will **NOT** die?
- This is it this is your time, how are you **SPENDING** it?

Here's how we **"dial-up"** our body's quadrillions of **"energy factories"** so we can perform at our absolute peak metabolic output.

Current Scenario of our Metabolically Sick Society (The Problem)

We spend billions of dollars every year buying:

- **Pills**
- **Potions**
- **Creams**
- **Injections**
- **Surgeries**

Why all this waste of time and money chasing an empty promise to slow the aging process? **What if** –as we slow the aging process and optimize healthy hair and beautiful skin – we took care of and trained our metabolism to help us live longer more healthy lives?

Meet your mitochondria

Mitochondria are micro power plants in our cells that convert the food (Substrates) we eat and the oxygen we breathe into ATP (ENERGY).

Mitochondrial, aging accelerates and performance declines, when the channel of communication between our cells is turned down- or off!

Here is the exciting news — the opposite is also true:

When communication is improved, the Aging process slows down, and overall health, **power**, **vitality** and general **function** improve when intracellular cellular communication is improved!

Modern science has stated that mitochondrial mutations were the reason we have age related intracellular cellular communication issues, but recent studies show that once poor communication issues- can be-repaired if not too advanced into decline.

"The aging process, we discovered, is like a married couple," states Harvard Medical School biologist David Sinclair, PhD. **"When they are young, they communicate well. But over time, living in close quarters for many years, communication breaks down."**

Fortunately, Sinclair notes: **"Restoring communication solves the problem."**

Caring for your mitochondria and upgrading their network of communication doesn't just slow down the aging process it can also enhance our:

- **Energy Metabolism (Physical Energy)**
- **Cognitive Powers (Mental Power)**

ARE YOU READY TO EMBARK ON A MITOCHONDRIAL MAKOVER?

Our premise at **M360** is: **WHAT IF!**

- What if we actually promoted our own health and sought to assist and improve our own cellular function, outside of a doctor's office and outside of the pharmaceutical confusion.
- What if we made a better effort to manage ourselves and seek to Bio Hack our own metabolic health- with better?
  - **Lifestyle decisions**
  - **Enjoyable physical activities**

- **Evidence based:**
  - ○ exercise
  - ○ nutrition
  - ○ stress management

Why Mitochondria Matter

What you need to know about your body's primary **SOURCE OF POWER!**

We would all be better off if we had a better understanding of the role of our mitochondria on our overall health!

Each one of us has quadrillions (that's thousands of trillions) of tiny power plants in the cells of our bodies. Each mitochondrion is filled with and estimated Seventeen Thousand biochemical assembly lines. Each assembly line is designed to produce ATP (molecule called adenosine triphosphate) — ATP is the Energy Currency of our Body. Like the $ dollar bill is the currency of our economy, **ATP is the "Currency" of Life! Powerful Stuff!**

The more energy a body part requires for proper optimal function, the more mitochondria the cells of that body part will contain. Mitochondria are very dense in cells that form and operate our:

- **Hearts**
- **Brains**
- **Muscles**

Up to 40% of the space in our Human **HEART** is taken up by mitochondrial power plants.

The health and density of our mitochondria within our organs and skeletal muscle is, to a large extent, a reflection of our current level of health and performance capacity. Our Lean Muscle Mass has far more mitochondria than our fat storage. It should also be noted that a strong heart is denser with mitochondria than a weak one.

Mitochondrial density in muscles and organs is a reflection of health and fitness, the more the better. Strong hearts will be very dense in mitochondria, much more so than weak ones.

- Our goal at M360 is a robust metabolism centered on a healthy landscape of mitochondria to drive optimal health and performance.
- The proliferation of healthy mitochondria equals more energy, focus, and optimal ability to sustain high levels of physical and mental activity without fatiguing.

Every step we take at **M360** is in support of mitochondrial health, from our exercise regimes to simple physical activities, recovery protocols and diets to **FEED** the **NEED** of our energy systems, our mitochondrial health and performance.

Mitochondria produce energy by breaking down and converting food into usable energy in the form of ATP (Energy Currency $ of the Human Body), along with some by-products, like carbon dioxide, water, and free radicals.

ROŞ (reactive oxygen species) also referenced as **Free radicals**, are highly charged, and active molecules that flow around the body, interacting with a variety of cells.

- **In moderation**, ROS can help us fight infection.
- Free radicals **In excess**, damage and erode our bodies- damaging cell tissue, and stimulating inflammation as well as accelerating *Pre Mature Aging!*

Mitochondria-related damage can be far-reaching. This damage can be held accountable for most of- if not **ALL** Chronic Disease.

Remember the math of our healthcare system?

$2.9 Trillion of $3.2 Trillion being spent on preventable, even reversible conditions! Anyone ever wonder why none of us mortal men can afford health insurance?

- **Bingo!** If insurance companies would adopt and support our **M360** programs the **Invoice for Healthcare** would be dramatically reduced.

Inactive lifestyles- paired with a poor selection of food and unchecked stress along with another can of sugar laden *"Energy Drink"* is simply destroying our energy systems. Why not correct our energy system once and for all -from the inside out? Education and evidence based, clinically correct —detailed and systematic path of execution- to better metabolic health is what we need.

The next Prescription your Healthcare Provider writes needs to be M360!

Much like **Drug REHAB**, we need a 8-12-week, 15-modality- **M36O** lifestyle program

- **Prescribed** by your healthcare provider,
- **Funded** in part by private insurance- and
- **Supported** by a complete test of biomarkers -before and after- the total immersion.

We must hold ourselves accountable to specific components of action driven by the explicit goal to optimize our metabolic fitness for life. We are the change, you and me!

Metabolic Fitness for Life!

What causes our mitochondria to deteriorate and our health to fail? The answer is that we eat a:

- **Excess of unhealthy foods** and a
- **Deficit of healthy ones**

Poor diets and lack of meaningful activity force mitochondria to burn through sugars, flours, and other processed foods— generating **EXCESSIVE** ROS, inflammation, and oxidation as they go. The result can be chronic conditions that lead to chronic disease.

Pro-inflammatory factors of high glycemic processed junk foods, trans-fats and chemical additives, increase cellular damage, unless we are eating plenty of:

- **Phytonutrients**
- **Sulforaphane**
- **Polyphenols**
- **Flavonoids**
- **Antioxidants**
- **Anti-Inflammatories**
- **Healthy Omega 3 fats**
- **Quality proteins**
- **Foods rich in fiber** (Soluble and Insoluble)
- **Foods containing Inulin**

You may be asking yourself as I have been asked, just what is a phytonutrient, or any other item on this list? **Short Answer** and **ALL** you need to concern yourself with at this point is that they are:

"A substance found in certain plants- which are believed to be beneficial to: human health, and the prevention of various diseases".

We are **NOT** giving our bodies what we need to repair and prevent ROS damage.

The epidemics listed below are the result of overfeeding and under nourishing our precious energy producing mitochondria:

- **Obesity**
- **Type 2 diabetes.**

When we overwhelm our pancreas with the production of too much insulin- the receptors in our cell membranes gradually become resistant to insulin reducing our ability to get what is needed into our mitochondria to produce energy. This is why we check for insulin resistance as one of our pre **M360** biomarker reference points.

From a genetic standpoint it is **CRITICAL** to understand, -that our mitochondria were *never* designed for the food and lifestyle that we currently expose them to. Unless we nurture and support our mitochondria, we will lose the optimal ability to perform at a variety of levels:

- **Elite Athletes** (Power)
- **Healthy Everyday People** (Vitality)
- **Active-Happy Senior citizens** (Function).

If we do not correct these issues we can develop a number of chronic diseases.

Understanding our mitochondria is critical in assisting them to perform for us, let's help them to convert the following into usable energy to fuel our healthy lives.

- **Food**
- **Oxygen**
- **ATP Energy**

When we eat unhealthy foods, and experience too much stress too often, we simply destroy our mitochondrial health. When **Free radicals** are produced in **EXCESS** we simply lose **Power, Vitality** and eventually **Function** to live.

How smart is it to destroy our source of Energy and Life?

Supporting our Life Giving, Mitochondrial Friends (The Solution)

We must adopt a more- **FAT ADAPTED** metabolism. Studies recommend avoiding foods containing gluten, processed lunch meats, and anything sweetened with sugar.

Basic wisdom recommends that we eliminate sugar laden foods and eat - 6 to 9 cups of vegetables and fruits daily to include:

- 3 green
- 3 deeply colored
- 3 rich in sulfur
- Research also recommends eating 6 to 12 ounces of grass-fed meat or wild-caught fatty fish daily.

At full force, our normally fat adapted diet becomes "ketogenic"

Ketogenesis forces fatty acids to enter the liver, to be broken down into "ketone bodies" that are in turn used for energy.

ATP production is enhanced and free-radical by-products are reduced when mitochondria are fueled by fat. Keep in mind every turn of the Krebs cycle produces 38 ATP from Sugar and a whopping 106 or more from Fat.

Functional Support of your Energy Systems

Help prevent and reverse mitochondrial decay. The best thing we can do to support our mitochondrial health is to eat a:

- **Organic**
- **Well-balanced**
- **Whole-Foods diet**

Definitive Ways to Improve Your Mitochondrial Function:

Caring for your mitochondria is the **KEY** to taking care of your health — and enjoying more **POWER, VITALITY, FUNCTION**, as well as increased- mental focus- in the process. We must be aware of this and focus our efforts in all 4 sections of this book toward optimal execution of: Lifestyle, Physical Activities, Exercise, Diet, Nutrition and Stress management. Our goal is Metabolic Fitness for Life!

Key Points of repairing and improving Metabolic Health for the Long Term:

- **Powerful Mitochondria through Reference Point Training:** Both endurance and resistance training can increase the number, and improve the function, of our mitochondria. The healthier our mitochondria, muscle mass and cardiovascular conditioning, the more Power, Vitality and Function we will have to achieve optimal health and improved performance.
- Processed flours, all sugars and refined sweeteners, trans-fats, gluten, and many: Non grass- fed dairy products are TOXIC to our mitochondria. **Avoid or eliminate these ingredients!**
- **Eat 6 - 9 cups of organic vegetables and fruits daily.** Choose from a variety of greens like
  1. Kale
  2. Broccoli,
  3. Spinach etc.
  4. Brightly colored vegetables beets, carrots, etc.
  5. Sulfur-rich (Sulforaphane) veggies (cauliflower, cabbage, etc.) these promote your metabolism to produce glutathione, a master antioxidant.

- **Dine on foods rich in complex fiber** which will assist your metabolism to detox poisons developed when mitochondrial function slows down.
- **Increase your consumption of omega-3 fats.** Omega 3 fats help to build up mitochondrial membranes. As a source of Omega 3 and quality protein M360 recommends the consumption of 6+ ounces of grass-fed meat, and/or wild-caught fish each day. Nuts, seeds and avocados are rich in quality fatty acids. M360 recommends that you consider supplementing 800 mg of EPA/DHA omega-3 daily.
- **Use Bone Broth in Cooking and as base broth for Soups.** There is increased risk for autoimmune diseases, such as arthritis, when mitochondria are compromised. These risks are caused, in part, by a **leaky gut**. Glutamine rich Bone broth and other amino acids can be especially good for healing a leaky gut along with other ailments. **Bone Broth** is the key ingredient in old-the Old School- chicken soup remedy.

Note: Damage to the lining of the small intestine is referred to as leaky gut, a condition which allows food particles to pass through the intestinal wall into our blood stream. Again: stress, poor diet and lifestyle choices are some of the leading causes of leaky gut. Correct the components of your lifestyle - improve diet, start effective physical activity and improving your management of stress is once **AGAIN** the solution.

- **Employ Probiotics and Fiber:**
  1. Probiotics are friendly bacteria in our gut, which bring about metabolically healthy benefits. Probiotics are living microorganisms.
  2. Prebiotics are non-digestible food ingredients that support our probiotic bacteria, and assist our Gut Flora/Micro biota. Non-soluble fiber (prebiotics) should be taken before and with probiotics to assist them in their live journey to our gut. Examples would be Chicory Root (rich in inulin),

Apples and Oatmeal. **M360** recommends a 50+ billion strain probiotic taken daily with plenty of soluble fiber. Dietary intervention to optimize gut micro biota is a solid nutritional strategy to improve:

- **Hypertension**
- **Lower Blood Pressure**
- **Excess Total Blood Cholesterol**

Research suggests that the **hypotensive** effects of **probiotics** may prove to be a promising intervention in the promotion of cardiovascular health.

Are sugary Packaged foods a part of your Lifestyle of Consumption? _____

Scientific facts are:

- The **Human Body** is designed to operate much more efficiently on a diet of **FAT** rather than a diet of **SUGAR**.
- My point here is for you to define and identify some of the obvious lifestyle traps you may have lying around your life, that keep you from success, by tripping you up.
  - **Sugar**
  - **Alcohol**
  - **Drugs**
  - **Cookies**
  - **Crackers**
  - **Soda Pop**
  - **Tobacco...**

When it comes to <u>SUGAR</u>- research is very clear:

- The more glucose your cells metabolize and the faster they do so, the more free radical oxidation occurs to damage DNA.

Once this occurs you leave yourself vulnerable to a cascade of metabolic events, which can potentially lead to Chronic Disease as a result of inflammation and oxidation.

- The simple description is when you eat sugar of all varieties and nonfiber (simple) carbohydrates, you will generate far more tissue damaging free radicals than when you burn (oxidize) body fat for fuel (energy).
- The more simple packaged carbohydrates and sugars- by any name- you consume- the more your pancreas secretes insulin and the cascade of events that follow can cause **Insulin Resistance** and more signals for your body to **STORE FAT!**

Remember the 2-Primary Functions of your metabolism are:

1. **Anabolism** or the **building up** and Storage of Fat (adipose tissue/body fat)
2. **Catabolism** or the **breaking down** of Fat Stores for use as energy (ATP)

<u>During anabolism</u> your cells are **uploading**:

- Sugar/glucose/carbohydrate- via **Insulin** secreted by your **Pancreas** into stores of **FAT** (Adiposity).
- Keep piling on the sugar/carbohydrate into your diet and you keep piling on layers of Fat as you **BURN OUT** the ability of your Pancreas to produce insulin, taken too far and you now have onset of **metabolic syndrome** or **type 2 diabetes,** along with a perfect environment for a variety of **chronic diseases.**

<u>During catabolism</u> your cells are **downloading**:

- Stores of body fat and using them to produce energy (ATP). The end sum of this **beautiful fat burning process** is you

○ **Reduce body fat and**
○ **Increase human energy** (ATP)

In a nutshell you start utilizing **FAT** for **FUEL**. We will specifically describe and prescribe things we can do in our programs of:

1. **Lifestyle Change**
2. **Exercise and Activity Execution**
3. **Diet Structure, Nutrition Quality and Nutraceutical Targets**
4. **Stress Management**

All efforts of our program point toward getting your metabolism running predominantly on Fat while reserving vital glucose stores for times they are most needed. Don't get me wrong, sugar is a lovely thing. Sugar is not a villain, the way we have abused it is!

For sake of keeping this book simple, I will assume that you, the reader would like to:

• **Reduce your fat storage**
• **Increase your lean mass**
• **Lower your overall body weight**
• **Increase Healthspan & Reduce Morbidity.**

Simple: We need to adapt your metabolism to burning **Fat for Fuel** rather that Sugar -Sugar -Sugar -**All the Time**. This is what we refer to as becoming:

FAT ADAPTED

Are you Metabolically Fat Adapted? _____

The goal of our book and program at **M360** is for you to fundamentally understand how your body works at a cellular, molecular and biological level. Although complex, in summary- it is very simple. If you learn nothing else, please understand the following paragraph:

We all have 2- Metabolic Pathways of converting food to energy:

1. **Sugar/Carbohydrate Metabolism** (glycolysis)
2. **Fat/Adiposity Metabolism** (lipolysis)

The descriptions of content in this section should start to clarify for you- the need to further:

- **LOWER** the **ACTIVATION** of your **Sugar Metabolism.**
- **INCREASE** the **ACTIVATION** of your **Fat Metabolism.**

The Prime goal of M360 is to become metabolically Fat Adapted!

It is often not just **HOW MUCH** you eat, but **WHAT** and **HOW OFTEN** you eat. All calories are **NOT** created equal.

- As you can see, *1-calorie of a sugar molecule* goes down an entirely different metabolic pathway than does, *1-calorie of a fat molecule.*

We will discuss in detail in section 2 and 3 a few methods of improving mitochondrial function and accelerate the transition from burning sugar to burning fat.

- **What is really enlightening** is the damage the sugar pathway (glycolic pathway) can cause with over oxidation (Free Radical Damage and Inflammation)
- **Show me excess Oxidation** and **Inflammation** and I will show you **Chronic Disease.**
- **Show me Chronic Disease** and I will show you a **Broken Healthcare System.** See my summary of conclusions at the end of the book for more.

What is "Classic" Inflammation?

Classic Inflammation- via our immune system is our body's first reaction to infection. Increased blood flow into the tissue visible by redness and swelling, are sure fired symptoms of inflammation. **Inflammation,** caused by bad eicosanoids and cytokines which are released by injured and infected cells.

Note: to keep it simple, **eicosanoids** and **cytokines** are signaling molecules. The cells of our body are amazing in their ability to interact and communicate both good and bad outcomes. Create inflammation with poor food choice, or reduce inflammation as a result of eating quality food and executing proper exercise and stress release. What can you do differently the next 16 hours of your life?

Inflammation is a survival mechanism against a hostile world

Inflammation is a defense mechanism against microbial attack and injury, without it we would have injuries that never heal. There are two different types of inflammation to be aware of:

1. Classic inflammation associated with pain, you can feel like a Bee Sting.
2. Chronic Silent inflammation that can go unnoticed as it occurs below the threshold of perceived pain.

What is "Silent" Inflammation?

Silent inflammation is something you cannot feel directly it can on for years (chronically), linger and wreak havoc on your entire metabolism, causing damage to:

- **Heart**
- **Brain**
- **Immune system**

Chronic- Silent Inflammation often leads to:

- **Heart disease**
- **Cancer**
- **Respiratory Disease**
- **Alzheimer's**

Inflammation is driven by hormones known as eicosanoids. Eicosanoids are made up of long-chain essential fatty acids that can be altered by **dietary interventions** (*nutraceuticals over pharmaceuticals*). Silent inflammation gets overlooked because it is there without you being able to feel it. Recent innovations in technology now allow us to measure silent inflammation with a new test referred to a hs- CRP or Cardio- CRP.

hs-CRP as a Clinical Biomarker of Chronic Inflammation and Oxidation

What is **high sensitivity C-Reactive Protein** (hs-CRP).

- C-reactive protein (CRP), as a response to inflammation, is produced by the liver in times of infection, and undue stress related to poor lifestyle choices and cellular injury.
- CRP is a key inflammatory biomarker -detected much faster than other markers of our blood.

hs-CRP is the first blood test you will do **BEFORE** our **M360**, 8-12- week 15- Modality program, and it is the first test we will take upon completion- as it is one of our 10- Biometric, Evidence Based Parameters- to Document Measurable Success.

What Causes Over Inflammation? It is all about Education & Choices!

What you choose to think, how you choose to react, how you choose to educate yourself about the function of your body, and how it reacts to choices you make. We all need to be in a **constant state of learning**. It is this philosophy that spawned our **Podcast on iTunes and Google Play "The Power 2 Learn"**. There is massive power in learning. **"We must Take it Upon Ourselves"** to always seek knowledge and learn!

One of my favorite sayings is:

WE simply do <u>NOT</u> know, what we do <u>NOT</u> <u>KNOW</u>, but we can change it!

What causes over inflammation in your body that leads to a cascade of events starting with inflammations buddy **"Oxidative Stress"**?

- How you **CHOOSE** to structure **LIFESTYLE?**
- How you **CHOOSE** to **EXERCISE?**
- What you **CHOOSE** to **EAT?**
- What you **CHOOSE** to **LEARN** and manage **STRESS?**

How do you breathe and react to what life-outside of your control throws at you?

M360 is about addressing **Oxidation** and **Inflammation** with every tool you have. How you think, how you exercise or execute your physical activities, what you eat, why, when and how with such simple things like how you breathe and learning the power to exhale and reduce stress.

We must arm ourselves with knowledge to make better choices?

Every day I see the insanity of people reacting to people, places and things- with the same limited response- expecting different outcomes, only to fail and be discouraged. **Don't be that person!**

We want you to pick **FOUR (4)** things to first be mindful of and then change, just **4** things, in your **16** waking hours, that you **<u>CAN-DO</u>** every single day to reduce: **Inflammation, Oxidation and with it... your proclivity toward Chronic Disease.**

Symptoms of inflammation include:

- **Overly Fat** Body Composition (Need Fat Adapted Metabolism)
- **Visible signs of Premature Aging** & wrinkles. (Reduce Oxidation/Inflammation)
- **Susceptibility to bacterial and viral infections**. (Need Probiotic)
- **Acid reflux** (Eliminate Simple Carbohydrates and Gluten)
- **Poor: Post Exercise Recovery Rate**. (Specific FFA Activities and Aerobic Transition Point (ATP) Training)
- **Poor Skin conditions and acne**. (Reduce Inflammation/ Oxidation)
- **Arthritis** (Reduce I/O)
- **Upper Respiratory Infections** (Auto Immune System)
- **Chronic pain** (Lower Inflammation with diet high in anti-inflammatories)
- **Pre Diabetic** (Reduce Sugar and balance Dietary Fat with Aerobic Activity)
- **High blood pressure** (nutraceuticals and ATP Exercise)
- **Osteoporosis** (50/70 Resistance Training)
- **Heart disease** (Lower HRV)
- **Candidiasis** (Nutraceuticals and FFA Training)
- **Urinary tract infections** (Nutraceuticals)

Chronic Inflammation is a gateway to Chronic Oxidative Stress

Chronic inflammation can be a major cause of cvd, cancer, copd and an increased rate of aging. Oxidative stress is induced by our Inflammatory process lowers our cellular antioxidant capacity.

What is Oxidative Stress and Free Radical Damage?

Oxidative Stress (OS) is an imbalance between the production of free radicals/Reactive Oxygen Species (ROS) and the ability of our body to detoxify the harmful effects- via neutralization with antioxidants. In a nutshell OS wins out and we age prematurely, over-oxidize, and put ourselves at greater risk of chronic disease.

Overproduction of free radicals can cause oxidative damage, eventually leading to many chronic diseases such as:

- **Atherosclerosis and other cardiovascular diseases**
- **Cancer**
- **Respiratory disease**
- **Diabetes**
- **Rheumatoid arthritis**
- **Stroke**
- **Septic shock**
- **Accelerated Aging and other degenerative diseases**

Oxidized LDL is atherogenic and is thought to be important in the formation of atherosclerosis plaques. Furthermore, oxidized LDL can directly damage endothelial cells (arterial walls), leading to blocked arteries.

Important to preface section 3 of this book where we will discuss in detail the idea of **"Nutraceuticals** over **Pharmaceuticals"**. In this example we would suggest whole organic foods that provide dietary nutraceutical antioxidants that provide B-carotene or vitamin E thus playing a vital and active role in the prevention of various cardiovascular diseases.

Imagine a healthcare system that supported education on nutraceutical food values over pharmaceutical dependencies and system breaking costs.

Shouldn't that be a wellness initiative of all Health Insurance Providers?

- How many people can benefit from our seminars and all inclusive clinically- biomarker based- 5 week intervention programs?
- Imagine what can we do with $2.9 Trillion Dollars?

Support **M360** to reduce and eliminate excessive healthcare costs, by educating and empowering, human performance, power, vitality and function at all levels.

What are symptoms of Oxidative Stress (OS)?

Because the free radicals resulting from oxidation- damage cells, proteins and our DNA (genes) and because OS itself is such a common process, the damage it can cause is significant. OS is known to cause:

- **Aging**
- **Grey hair**
- **Wrinkles**
- **Arthritis**
- **Decreased eye sight**
- **Cancer**

So, how can you tell if oxidative stress is occurring in your body?

1. **Fatigue**
2. **Memory loss and/or brain fog**
3. **Muscle and/or joint pain**
4. **Wrinkles and grey hair**
5. **Decreased eye sight**
6. **Headaches and sensitivity to noise**
7. **Susceptibility to infections**

HOW M360 gets at reducing OXIDATIVE STRESS

M360 programs will always present programs of **ACTION**:

- Seminars
- Podcast's
- Exercise sessions
- Lifestyle coaching
- Stress management
- Intervention sessions
- Meal preparation classes

M360 Programs will always present and act upon the latest research in reducing the underlying factors of our mortality and performance.

M360 is not about one person preaching, it is about a community of like minded learners, seeking knowledge on common topics, which will change our health and wellness outcomes.

There is massive power in grouping like minded seekers of truth, hungry to improve and excel at life- rather than, isolate, stagnate and deteriorate alone.

There are two ways to reduce oxidative stress:

- Avoiding exposure to unnecessary oxidation
- Increasing endogenous and exogenous anti-oxidants at the cellular level.

Decreasing Exposure to Oxidation

Oxidative Stress (OS) increases when we are exposed to stress, toxins, and infections. It is also increased by **sugar** and chemicals, so the more you can minimize your exposure to these things, the better – so choosing organic foods and avoiding toxins in your environment makes a big difference. Reducing stress helps too and can be done with what I refer to as **"moment to moment- stress remedies"** like breathing. No need to wait, you can do it **RIGHT NOW!**

Breathing Exercise to reduce Stress

STOP... bring all of your attention to your wave of breathing—**IN** and **OUT**... slowly and deeply inhale as you focus, relax and fully **EXHALE!** Feel the depth of your exhalation and **RELAX**- release-focus and flow around your exhalation.

Notice how the more you **EXHALE** the **DEEPER** you will **INHALE**. Practice this -continuous wave flow- as need be and let go of the unnecessary stress you are lugging around.

We will discuss chronic disease, oxidative stress and inflammation in each section as they apply to exercise, diet, and stress management.

Each word of **M360** is meant as a reference to our program. This is **NOT** a novel. Feel free to pick and choose sections to read as they apply to what it is you are looking to biohack, or alter in your own program. We would be remiss to not cover:

The Basics of Hormonal Balance and Health

1. Insulin – The Fat Storing hormone

Insulin is #1 when it comes to hormonal influence on fat loss! Insulin is influenced by:

- **Carbohydrate intake**
- **Unchecked Stress**
- **Over consumption of food**

Combinations of any of these in excess- will cause detrimental increases in blood sugar levels!

Over consuming Protein, Carbohydrate, and Fat can elevate insulin levels.

- Sedentary, over-consumers, insulin levels will increase and remain high.
- Over production of insulin can cause your body to become resistant and you will have difficulty utilizing fat as a fuel substrate.
- There is an epidemic of type II diabetes and obesity. **M360** will ask you to take an Insulin Resistance test which will provide a number (IR-Score) from 1-100 with 1 being insulin sensitive, and 100 being **Insulin Resistant**. Insulin resistant means you are <u>**UNABLE**</u> to burn/utilize fat. **With lots of insulin around you cannot burn fat! Our prime objective is to shift your metabolism from sugar addicted to FAT ADAPTED and with it get your IR Score in line with Metabolic Fitness for Life**
- **Insulin Resistance** is one of the key biomarkers we will be targeting with lifestyle change, shifts in diet and adaptations to exercise and stress relief.

The magic of M360 comes as your metabolism shifts into a fat adapted mode- moving away from insulin resistance and becoming more and more insulin sensitive, thus relieving metabolic stress and the negative cascade of events that follow.

2. Glucagon – The Fat Burner

Glucagon and Insulin- in a healthy body, work together, to keep your blood sugar and energy requirements balanced.

- Higher levels of glucagon in our body **enable us to burn fat instead vs. storing it**. When insulin levels are low- glucagon will be produced to assist our bodies to burn fat for fuel.
- The key to increased glucagon production is to minimize carbohydrate intake and refrain from over-eating.
- We will also utilize:

1. **FFA** Training (FFA)
2. **ATP** Training (ATP)
3. **Sub Lactate Threshold** (LBP)/(HIIT)
4. **Intermittent Fasting** (IF)
5. **Time Restricted Eating Specific to Your Life** (TRE)

All arrows of effort point toward vastly improve Fat Utilization to develop a strong **Fat Adapted Metabolism** and **Metabolic Fitness for Life!**

3. Ghrelin – Referred to as the "Hunger Hormone"

Because Ghrelin increase in the body when you are physically hungry, it is called the hunger hormone.

Note: There is a big difference between physical hunger, and emotional hunger, we must make the effort to identify and understand the difference. Being better aware of this situation will help us to significantly impact fat loss.

4. Thyroid Hormone – The Metabolic Manager

Thyroid hormones (TH) regulate our metabolism and help to manage our metabolic processes including our **fat burning capacity**. Thyroid hormones are very in-tune with the components of our lifestyle including:

- **Sleep**
- **Nutrition**
- **Stress**
- **Exercise**

5. Cortisol – The Stress Hormone

Cortisol is secreted from our adrenal glands, and has a duel personality -it is not all bad or all good. Acute stressors on the body can stimulate short-term increases of cortisol.

- Cortisol will primed our body to either fight or flee from stress. When we were not at the top of the food chain. A wild animal attack required a metabolic alarm to prime us to fight or flee. When this situation of danger passed Cortisol had the power to stimulate Growth Hormone to assist us in recovery and make us stronger for the next time a danger presented itself.
- In modern time, technical times- our lifestyles have become so distorted and full of noise that our adrenal glands think we are surrounded by dangerous creatures and threats of danger everywhere, this causes our cortisol levels to swing from very high, to very low; both of which create a fatty, fatigued body.
- Cortisol released with HGH (human growth hormone) and testosterone can become a fat burning influencer.

To stimulate the production of positive Cortisol hormone we should exercise in three (3) prime modalities, or reference points, what we will detail as Reference Point Training (RPT) in Section 2:

1. **Long duration** low intensity, what we call Free Fatty Acid (FFA) Training in an Unfed State at general intensities of **45-75%** of Max Heart Rate (MHR). Duration can vary from 1-hr walk to 8 hour 100 mile bike ride.
2. **Medium Intensity** Aerobic Transition Point (ATP) Training also in an Un-Fed State, with emphasis on Sustainable POWER **75-85%** of MHR. Duration will vary from 20 minute to 90 minute at peak ATP output. Often referred to as a "TEMPO" session.
3. **Short duration** -higher intensity interval training (HIIT), movements, with the primary focus on 2-20 minute efforts

between **85-90%** of MHR. The key here is coming up to and just above- and below Onset of Blood Lactate Accumulation (OBLA). Another word for OBLA is Lactate Threshold or (LT) or Lactate Balance Point (LBP). In terms of **M360** we will emphasis a small amount of this intensity and pay extra attention to keeping effort below LT.

One problem with today's fitness industry is:

- **Too much intensity**
- **Too often**
- **Not enough endurance base FFA/ATP to support it**

The result is much like sugar, too much -too often only creates more **Metabolic Acidosis, Oxidative Stress, Inflammatory Response** and **General stress** leading to overtraining, illness and injury, whilst missing the true body building aspects of improving the human Fat Metabolism- Power, Vitality and Function at ATP based on expanded Aerobic Capacity and a healthy metabolism.

Nutraceutical Intervention with Functional Whole Food

Nutrition is incredibly important to the prevention of chronic diseases, with most chronic disease being related to diet. Functional Whole Food is not only necessary for metabolic life to thrive, functional foods rich in Nutraceuticals provide a source of mental and physical well-being, that contribute to the reduction and prevention of several diseases that will bring us down psychologically as well as physiologically.

Food is considered functional when it benefits one or more metabolic functions within our body, functions relevant to our health and performance as well as our state of well-being and the reduction and risk of a disease.

Examples of Functional Whole Foods with specific Nutraceutical value:

- Tomatoes, Carrots, and Broccoli are functional foods because of their Nutraceutical components of (sulforaphen, B-carotene, and lycopene, respectively).
- Green Vegetables
- Spices like mustard and turmeric, also can fall under this category.

"Nutraceutical" is a term coined in 1979 by Stephen De Felice. He defined it as:

"A food, or parts of food, that provide medical or health benefits, including the prevention and treatment of disease."

Nutraceuticals have scientifically proven health benefits for both the treatment and prevention of disease. As I did the research for this writing, it was just amazing how powerful the ingredients of plants can be. Key nutraceutical ingredients in plants are flavonoids, which act as potent antioxidants. Flavonoids are recognized to possess anti-inflammatory, antiviral, and anticarcinogenic benefits. You are missing the boat if you are not consuming a variety of quality organic plants at some level!

We will further discuss this in section 3.

Just a few ingredients that make food functional are:

- **Dietary fibers**
- **Vitamins**
- **Minerals**
- **Antioxidants**
- **Essential fatty acids** (omega-3)
- **Bacteria cultures**

Many of these are present in medicinal plants. Indian systems of medicine believe that complex diseases can be treated with complex combinations of botanicals unlike in our western culture, with single drugs.

Some medicinal plants with powerful nutraceutical function are spices such as:

- **Onion**
- **Garlic**
- **Mustard**
- **Red chilies**
- **Turmeric**
- **Clove**
- **Cinnamon**
- **Saffron**
- **Curry**
- **Ginger**

Whether it is organizing your lifestyle, exercising, physical activities or nutritional selections, your **CHOICE** always has an **EFFECT** on your metabolism. Our goal is to work together to make better decisions leading to sustainable metabolic fitness for life.

A Healthy Metabolism is your Source of Life and Fountain of Youth!

The very word Metabolism is from the Greek *Metabole* meaning "Change". Everything we breathe and consume is processed by our metabolism to **generate and regenerate life.** How well you can generate and regenerate life is our Fountain of Youth. When we chose the title of this book and our program we fell in love with Metafit.life, not only as a web domain, but as a brand. The name says it all:

Metabolic Fitness for Life! (M360 for short)

The sole goal of our program is to get our readers, podcast listeners and program members- to understand basics of the human metabolism and how our bodies generate energy. We want each reader to understand the products and by-products produced by our human energy systems or metabolism. There are many things we can do to **SUPPORT** it and many things we can do to **SABOTAGE** it. The course you take often depends on **MAKING** time to learn how your metabolism works. Let's take a look at the basics.

Metabolic Pathways of Energy Production

Human Energy is critical to the vitally of your life, your power output on a bike, your speed as a runner, swimmer or athlete in general. Human Energy is critical to your endurance for work, play and life. Without the ability to produce **ENERGY**, you have **NOTHING!**

Million Dollar Question: How well do you produce ENERGY- ATP?

We defined the organic chemical known as ATP or Adenosine Triphosphate in earlier pages as the energy currency of the human body that is found in **ALL** forms of life on our planet! Our bodies produce roughly our own body weight equivalent in ATP each day. ATP is also a foundation to our DNA and RNA. Pretty lofty stuff my friend!

ATP is the molecular currency of intracellular energy transfer in our precious bodies.

ATP Fuels our Life!

ATP is LIFE! ATP dictates your work capacity, vitality, power, ability to function, and endurance to sustain. Without ATP we cease to exist!

How do you structure your day to optimize your metabolic health and ATP production via mitochondrial health?

At this point you must know the structure of **M360** is to get you to take it upon yourself to optimize the structure of your life, this is your lifestyle. Optimize it to the point that your allocate time to sleep properly, eat properly, exercise and relax properly and promote metabolic fitness at the mitochondrial level. Research indicates that mitochondria account for about 10% of your body weight, approximately 10 million – Billion mitochondria cells in average adults.

What is Mitochondrial Health?

We now know that mitochondria are the power plants of our cells. We plan to improve your health one cell at a time, in fact- your health is how well you function as a human being at the: **Cellular Level.**

What is your mitochondrial state of health?_____

Mitochondria are continuously producing ATP adenosine triphosphate. Every cell of our body needs a continuous supply of energy 24/7 to sustain life. To simplify my point there are two major biological processes needed to meet energy requirements:

- **Eating**
- **Breathing**

What you eat, how often you eat, and how efficient you breathe- are huge factors of your health- you have more control over than you may think.

The purpose of M360 is to get you to dig deeper into the simple routines you can adopt in your life to bring enormous change to the quality of your life. For example, if you learn how to make the following part of your day:

- **Eating no sooner to bedtime than 3 hours, or simply:**
- **Not eating for a 14-16 hour intermittent period of time from day to day you can dramatically:**

1. **Reduce your body fat content**
2. **Adapt your metabolism to utilize body fat for fuel/ energy.**
3. **Lower inflammation and oxidation.**

Make these ideas- actions in your life and you will completely change your health and wellness landscape. **You can alter:**

- **Longevity**
- **Health Span**
- **Dramatically improve the way you FEEL**

In light of a modern media driven landscape of ridiculous diets and brutal "Whoop -Whoop Go Girl", or "Hey Dude Boot Camps" you can find the truth.

The Metabolic Truth to better Fat Adaption, more meaningful exercise/ activity and a simple diet that will provide delicious healthy anti-oxidant foods that assists your body in this enormous lifelong metabolic process of creating energy and eliminating waste as it deals with Oxidation or "Rusting". Put a shine on your health; help your little mitochondrial friends out.

Just as ATP is the Molecular Energy Currency of your Life, your Lifestyle is the Framework of your Life. How do you Position or FRAME Nutrition and Activity or Diet and Exercise to Optimize and Sustain Energy?

Everything we frame and position with our **M360 LIFESTYLE** must support metabolic fitness and mitochondrial function. We must frame proper exercise and nutrition to support our organism at a cellular level. When people ask me about their health and human performance I always look at them and try to imagine the internal landscape of their cells. What does it look like in there?

Are you high or low in Oxidative Stress?_____

Oxidative stress is an imbalance between the systemic creation of reactive oxygen species (ROS), and our metabolic ability to detoxify and repair the resulting damage.

Oxidative stress was first defined as:

A cellular disturbance of pro-oxidant vs. antioxidant balance in favor of Oxidation

Like an apple turns brown when exposed to air, our cells can "rust" when we breathe due to **oxidative stress**, a process **caused** by free radicals.

All things Oxidative Stress

Endothelial cells line our vascular walls throughout our entire circulatory system, from our heart to the smallest capillaries. Oxidative stress is linked to cardiovascular disease, because oxidation of LDL in the vascular wall is strongly linked to plaque formation. This cascade of events includes both strokes and heart attacks and general poor performance in a variety of disciplines.

Oxidative stress has also been associated with chronic fatigue syndrome. Oxidative stress can contribute overall cellular injury (aging) as well as promote the onset of diabetes and disease of our respiratory system.

Oxidative stress is also associated with the age-related development of cancer. ROS production from oxidative stress has the potential to cause direct damage to DNA and further increase reactive oxygen species in our stomach linking OS to the development of gastric cancer.

Food based nutraceutical agents are capable of scavenging and removing ROS species from our systems.

- **Glutathione** is an example of an antioxidant that is endogenously produced along with agents found in our diet- such as ascorbic acid (Vitamin C and vitamin E).

Are you getting enough vitamin C and vitamin E?_____

Numerous dietary antioxidants may also contribute to cellular protection against radicals and other ROS. Important dietary antioxidants include vitamin E, vitamin C, and **carotenoids.** Vitamin E is one of the most widely distributed antioxidants in nature, and it is the primary chain-breaking antioxidant in cell membranes.

NOTE: What is a Carotenoid?

Plant pigments known as Carotenoids, are responsible for bright colors of many vegetables and fruits.

Caratanoids serve an important role in the health of plants that we eat. When we eat these plants we get these same nutraceutical values.

Carotenoids are considered phytonutrients, or plant chemicals that are rich in polyphenols and flavonoids. Carotenoids are found in the cells of plants, algae and bacteria. Carotenoids provide the antioxidant function of deactivating free radicals (ROS).

Do you EAT a Plant Based Diet full of COLOR and rich in Carotenoids?

Intermittent Fasting and Autophagy (cellular cleansing)

Studies suggest that basal **autophagy** has the potential to clear out potentially harmful metabolic aggregates associated with the onset of chronic disease.

Autophagy is activated during periods of nutrient deprivation and cellular starvation. Autophagy is thought to play a key role in our anti-aging mechanisms of caloric-restriction.

Research supports the theory that -**caloric-restriction**- can reduce and even prevent age-dependent detrimental changes in cells with an increased frequency of autophagy. *See Power 2 Learn Podcast on Autophagy

Diet and Inflammation

The connection between diet and inflammation reside in the immune system. Our immune system is highly sensitive to the foods and nutrients we provide it. The inflammatory response is based on the condition of our immune system and WHAT we choose to feed it. This is why our diet is intimately associated with our regulation of silent inflammation. Dietary selections can activate the inflammatory response or inhibit it. Which one do you choose to associate yourself with?

Clinical Markers of Silent Inflammation

Until **NOW** it has been difficult to discuss the topic of silent inflammation because it typically has no pain associated with it. It could not be measure- so it remained silent- but deadly inflammation, however now we have new measurable clinical markers of silent inflammation in the form of a simple blood test- called high-sensitivity C-reactive protein (hs-CRP or Cardio CRP).

What are the Dietary Origins of Silent Inflammation?

- **Increased consumption of refined carbohydrates**
- **Increased consumption of refined vegetable oils rich in omega-6 fatty acids**
- **Decreased consumption of long-chain omega-3 fatty acids**

Increased consumption of refined carbohydrates significantly increases the glycemic load of our diet. The glycemic load of what we eat is defined as the amount of carbohydrate that is consumed multiplied by the glycemic index of what you ate.

High glycemic-index carbohydrates are the key ingredient in virtually all processed foods:

- Potato
- Rice
- Bread products
- White Flour Tortillas

The cost of refined carbohydrates has decreased dramatically, while at the same time the availability to produce products with these ingredients has dramatically increased.

Increasing the consumption of high glycemic- refined food products results in the increased secretion of insulin resulting in the ever increasing postprandial rise of blood glucose. Simply put your blood sugar levels 2 hours after a meal go higher and higher till they reach dangerous levels.

What is Bad Fat?

Increased insulin production can only explain a portion of the rapid increase in silent inflammation. Bad fats are the other dietary component that destroys our metabolism:

- Cheap vegetable oils rich in omega-6 fatty acids have bombarded the market.
- Omega-6 fatty acid known as linoleic acid is the primary fatty acid in the most vegetable oils. Read the Label

It is only in the last 50 years that linoleic acid has become a regular component of our human diet.

- Fats that contain less than 10% linoleic acid such as butter, lard, and olive oil are not as widely used as they once were.
- Cheap vegetable oils contain 50%–75% linoleic acid. Such oils come from corn, soy, sunflower, and safflower.
- Cheap vegetable oil consumption has increased more than 400% since 1980.
- With the combination of these two dietary trends -refined carbohydrates and vegetable oils- there should be NO surprise over the dramatic increase in silent inflammation. **Remember:** Show me Inflammation and Oxidation and I will show you Chronic Conditions that lead to Chronic Disease!

NOTE: A steady diet of refined carbohydrate, paired with the increased consumption of vegetable oils rich in linoleic acid, will increase silent inflammation.

Anti-Inflammatory Diet Based on Anti-Inflammatory Nutrition

Anti-inflammatory nutrition starts with understanding how individual nutraceuticals affect our metabolism. The first step to sustaining an anti-inflammatory diet would be to execute the nutrient considerations described above, as well as being sustainable for a lifetime.

A good diet starts with the 30,000 ft view of 3-Macronutrients in a balance that will promote a Fat Adapted Metabolism.

Dietary Fat (50%-70% of Sample 2,000 Calorie Diet)

Health authorities and the media have been bombarding us with misinformation about fats for far too many years, promoting low-fat diets, while advising us to avoid foods like coconut oil and butter.

Modern research now contradicts the nutritional myth that fats – saturated fats, in particular – are bad for us. Our first mistake was increasing refined carbohydrate and reducing good fat. This only promotes sugar addiction and reduces fat adaption which will increase inflammation and oxidation. Crazy Stuff my Friend!

Endogenous man has eaten animal products for the majority of our time on earth. Endogenous man/woman kinds were hunter-gatherers consuming diets abundant in meats and plants. From an evolutionary perspective- suggesting that saturated fats are suddenly harmful to us is really an insult to our intelligence or ability to discern.

Dietary Fat is Very Important (Healthy)

Healthy **Saturated fats** are found in products like:

- **Butter**
- **Cheese**
- **Whole raw milk**
- **Fatty meats.**

It is important to do your own label and content research and discern against various good and bad fats -hydrogenated vegetable, seed oils, which have been artificially modified into saturated fats. Known as *trans* fats these fats can interfere with our insulin receptors and launch a cascade or metabolic events that lead to chronic diseases like cancer, heart disease and diabetes.

A flawed study by an influential and misguided scientist, Dr. Ancel Keys, is the reason saturated fats have been demonized. Mr. Keys mistakenly linked higher saturated fat intake to higher rates of heart disease. Saturated fat found naturally in animal and plant sources is not the villain –it's the *trans* fats you need to concern yourself with found in:

- **Margarine**
- **Vegetable Shortening**
- **Partially hydrogenated vegetable oil**

Sources of healthy dietary fat

Animal fats containing beneficial levels of omega-3s are a great fat source. Recent Studies position healthy fats from these sources to comprise of anywhere from *50 to 70% of your overall energy intake*. With that said fats are also the most caloric macronutrient by volume, so make sure that at least half of your dinner plate is still taken up with plant based food.

What Really Makes our Modern Society so FAT?

Our society has always promoted food high in complex-carbohydrate and low in saturated fats with healthy high-fat foods perceived as a health risks.

Healthy Benefits of fat:

Over consuming sugar and processed grain can lead to neural impairment and cellular damage, and interfere with insulin signaling. Consuming healthy fats as your prime fuel substrate is crucial to your brain function. Without fats our brain cannot function.

Optimal brain health is dependent on essential Omega-3 fats to function properly. Very few people get enough Omega -3 through diet alone, omega-3 deficiency is linked to as many as 96,000 premature deaths every year.

The perfect recipe for silent inflammation and chronic disease is to:

- Eat too many inflammatory omega-6 fats (like cheap vegetables oils)
- Eat too few anti-inflammatory omega-3 fats.

HOW MUCH Protein?

Protein consumption should be between 20–30 grams at every meal. This would be enough to increase thermogenesis and activate protein synthesis in most of us. In terms of meat this would be 3-4 grams of quality meat, fish or poultry. Feed the Need.

What is dietary Thermogenesis?

The thermic (Thermogenic) effect of food (TEF) is referred to as **dietary induced thermogenesis** (DIT). DIT is the metabolic amount of energy our body will spend to digest food into a usable form for our metabolism to store or utilize.

Example: let's say an apple is 100 calories, but it takes your body 50 calories of energy to break it down and digest. This would be a net caloric consumption of 50 calories at a thermogenic cost of 50 calories. Consider the thermogenic effect of eating an apple vs. drinking a 12 ounce glass of apple juice. Which one has a higher **"Thermogenic Effect"**? The Apple of course has a much greater thermic effect, as it cost your body more to break down or digest into a usable substrate. Keep thermogenesis in mind as we present our dietary program in section 3.

Protein (20%-30% of Sample 2,000 Calorie Diet)

Amino acids found in protein are the building blocks of our hormones, enzymes, muscles, and bones. We cannot live without protein.

Can you eat *too much* protein? The answer is- **YES and Most of us Do!**

Excessive Protein Intake

We typically eat far more protein than we need- which increases our glycemic load, especially as we are generally do so along with high glycemic- refined carbohydrates- and not enough healthy fats.

Too much protein can be detrimental to your metabolic health:

- **Elevating blood glucose levels**
- **Promoting weight gain**
- **Storing extra body fat**
- **Stressing your kidneys**
- **Leaching important bone minerals and**
- **Causing dehydration**

Protein consumption is a game of moderation where more is not better. Meet your body's needs with the use of adequate levels to meet your bodies' metabolic needs, more on this in section 3 on feeding the need.

Vegetarian/Vegan Diets and Health

To get sufficient protein intake it is necessary to mix a combination of plant and animal sources. **M360** does not recommend a strict vegetarian or vegan diet. As there are many nutrients that cannot be obtained from plant foods, it is wise to mix in a moderate amount of animal products to insure a balanced diet.

Daily Protein Requirement

How much protein do you need? What do you do? How hard do you do it? What is your **lean body mass (LM)** or **fat free mass (FM)**.

Start with one-half gram of protein per pound of lean body mass.

If you are 100 pounds at 30% body fat, you are 70 pounds lean and 30 pounds fat. ½ a gram of protein per lean pound would dictate a starting point of 35 grams for our example. If we are training very hard for a competition, our protein requirement may be 30 to 60 percent higher.

This is why Our Motto is:

Feed the Need specific to who you are- and what you do! Anabolic and Catabolic states are fed differently. We will expand on this in section 3 of this book and in our Podcast's at *Power 2 Learn* on iTunes and Google Play.

The message here is to better understand Anabolic and Catabolic Metabolic States. If you spend the day watching television, which is perfectly fine on occasion you may consume half a gram of protein per pound of lean mass. Using myself for example this would be half of 160 pounds LM. So I would consume 80 grams in the course of the day 20-30 grams at a time. If I lifted real heavy after a 50 mile bike ride I may consume as much as 160 grams or 1 gram per pound of LM. **Feed the NEED!**

Calculating your lean body mass

- Subtract your percent body fat from 100.
- 20 percent body fat, then you have 80 percent lean body mass
- To get your lean body (**LM**) mass in pounds multiply lean mass percentage (in this case, 0.8) by your current weight.
- Our sample is 160 pounds, so I would multiply that amount by 0.8 (representing 80 percent) which leaves you with 128 pounds of lean body mass, with a 32 pound fat mass (FM)
- Starting point for protein at "1/2 gram of protein per pound of lean mass" rule, you would need about 64 grams of protein per **low activity** day- up to 128 grams (1 gram per lb/LM) on a highly intense activity day.

I recommend that you write down everything you eat for a few days or simply connect your Garmin Connect Activity Tracker to myfitnesspal. com) **See Section 2 &3 of this book**

Source and Quality of Protein Matters

Grass Fed meat is a great source of protein but there are other great foods with substantial amounts of protein to consider:

- **Wild Caught Fish**
- **Range Free Poultry**
- **Wild Meats**
- **Nuts**
- **Seeds**

Egg Protein

Eggs protein provides the required 8-essential amino acids. Our choice of eggs are true free-range eggs, which come from hens allowed to roam freely outdoors that consume a natural diet of seeds, worms, insects, and green plants. Eggs from free ranging hens contain superior nutrient levels:

- **Two-thirds more vitamin A**
- **Three times more vitamin E**
- **Two times more omega-3 fatty acids**
- **Seven times more beta carotene**

Soft-boiled is the best cooking option, while *Scrambled or fried eggs can oxidize the cholesterol in the eggs and ruin the value of your meal.*

Carbohydrate (10%-20% of Sample 2,000 Calorie Diet)

Focusing on fats and not carbs will be a very important part of the **M360** plan. When we talk carbohydrates we are talking -**net carbs**- defined as: total carbs minus fiber. This is **NOT** a low **TOTAL** carb diet, but rather- a low **NET** carb diet. **M360** recommends fibrous carbs in your diet for two primary reasons. As a prebiotic which is beneficial to probiotic bacteria, and the metabolic use of fiber as it is converted to short chain fats to be used for energy other than sugar.

Facts on Fiber

- Fiber affects: Digestion, heart, and skin health, improved blood sugar levels, weight management, and more.
- Vegetables, some fruits, nuts, and seeds are the most healthful sources of fiber not whole grains!
- M360 recommends 50 grams of fiber per 1,000 calories. Average Americans get nowhere near this amount.

Burning carbs as your primary fuel is a problem - carbs do not burn as cleanly as fat and are known to produce 30% to 40% more (ROS) than fat.

The goal of **M360** is to limit your intake of net carbs to fewer than 40 to 50 grams per day for a given period and fill in those calories with healthy fats, these steps will transition your body into burning fat for fuel rather than sugar while reducing your proclivity toward chronic disease.

Let Your IR Scores Dictate Your Ongoing Carb Intake

Know your I/R Score — *this is part of the NMR Panel we will require before you begin our M360 program.* The test will provide information on where you are in terms of an insulin scale from **"Insulin Sensitive on the left at 0 to Insulin Resistant on the right at 100"**. I personally was at **<24** on a few recent tests, which is good. I also test my post prandial (after meal) reaction to food with a glucose meter, so I have a good idea how my metabolism is reacting to the food I consume.

Wherever you are- our goal with **ALL** actions of **M360** is to **Optimize and Document Standard Biomarkers** of your long term sustainable health and performance.

Insulin regulates blood sugar levels. Insulin is secreted when you eat high glycemic loads. Excessive eating of any food even excessive protein, can lead to insulin resistance.

If your insulin resistance test result (I-R Score) is below 35, then your carbohydrate consumption may be ideal specific to your own metabolism. If the levels are higher, then you must cut back or eliminate grain starches and sugars from your diet. **You must take it upon yourself to know your insulin resistance score (I-R Score), the higher the score the less carbohydrates you should eat.**

What is your Insulin Resistance Score (IR Score)?

If you're already insulin resistant you need to lower total net carbohydrates below 50g for a time and let your body spend some time seeking out stored fat as your prime metabolic energy substrate.

Organic Vegetables

As you wean yourself off sugar and refined carbohydrate you need to transition your meals to reflect a diet rich in colorful fresh, organic raw vegetables and some fruits like avocado. Fibrous- carbohydrates that will improve your metabolic health, and reduce Oxidative Stress while providing your cells with bioavailable-nutraceutical vitamins, nutrients, and minerals.

Variety of vegetable, fruits, nuts and meats is the key to overall nutrient balance. Check out our blog at www.metafit.life for updates and ideas.

HOW you prepare vegetables is important. Heat can strip some vegetables of nutrients and expose nutrients for others. For the most part however it is best to eat vegetables **RAW**. We will have ongoing meal preparation classes at **M360** as part of our program. Eating is a blessing and the preparation of quality foods can be very enjoyable and a lot of **FUN**.

Seek out vegetables with the highest content of polyphenols and the least amount of carbohydrates. Eat colorful, nonstarchy, vegetables, with moderate amounts of fruit. Low glycemic plant based meals, with moderate amounts of quality protein, will reduce inflammation and oxidation.

Lifestyle Timing and Adaptation to a Natural Rhythm

M360 simply proposes that we get in-line with our natural rhythm and routine, and that we qualify what we:

- Do in terms of work, activity and exercise.
- What we choose to feed our metabolic need in terms of nutrition.
- How we manage our stress in the 16 waking hours we have each day.

We have a <u>MASSIVE</u> opportunity to improve and support our metabolic function each and every 24 hour cycle. M360 is all about intervention and adaptations to assist and optimize metabolic function at every level of activity, nutrition and mindset possible.

Optimizing our metabolic health is partially a matter of doing a better job of dialing up healthy and natural circadian rhythms. We must incorporate our physiology and psychology to coordinate metabolic function and behavior into robust daily patterns or biological rhythms.

Feeding, fasting, physical activity, stress management and specific exercise must all come together to optimize our being, our health and our ability to perform. When it comes to eating, or feeding it is not so much a matter of what we eat, as it is a matter of **WHEN** and **HOW**

OFTEN. Feeding is a balanced metabolic cycle we need to optimize and better align ourselves with.

M360 Metabolic Health and Dietary patterns

Our anti-inflammatory diet in a sample volume of 1,995 calories per day would consist of roughly:

- 155 grams of good fat (1,395 calories) 70%
- 100 grams of quality protein (400 calories) 20%
- 50 grams of low glycemic - high fiber net carbohydrates (200 calories) 10%

This sample represents a balance of **70%** good dietary fat, **20%** quality dietary protein, and **10%** quality plant based, dietary and **Fibrous Net Carbohydrates**. Once you become more fat adapted and- I must add, much more active, and we see our biomarkers improving, this dietary structure may shift to 50% fat, 20-25% protein and more carbohydrates at 15-30%.

Don't worry you have not eaten your last piece of cake or other sweet delight. We will show you the massive benefits of dark chocolate, apples, blueberries and other decadent delights that are very good for you.

Feed the Need by getting in Biological Rhythm with WHAT we DO!

Protein requirements are necessary to maintain a positive nitrogen balance and supply enough essential amino acids for optimal metabolic function, growth and repair.

Please note that higher levels of exercise in either the Male or Female would require still higher protein intakes to compensate for the catabolism of muscle occurring during more intense strength and power training. This increase would also bump up total calories in correlation with the increase in protein - more on this in Section 3.

The **M360** anti-inflammatory food plan- does not include bread and grains (especially refined grain products). M360 total calories come from the consumption of bright colorful vegetables and some fruits (i.e., rich in polyphenols). This shift into plant based calories has a significant hormonal response that leads to a lower and lower inflammatory stress response. How do we know? Cardio CRP levels with go down!

Weight loss is **NOT** the goal of our **M360** anti-inflammatory diet. Fat adaption and a Reduction of silent inflammation is our target. Weight/ Fat loss however is a positive side effect. **Note:** Silent inflammation is the key to increased body fat in the first place. **M360 will reduce body fat by reducing inflammation.**

The success of our anti-inflammatory **M360** diet will be clinically documented by our various biomarkers of silent inflammation that we will test before and after your **M360** Immersion Block. We will also targeting your Insulin Resistance (IR Score) and post exercise recovery rates (PERR).

The Power of Intermittent Fasting (IF) and Time Restricted Eating (TRE):

Intermittent fasting is simply going a short duration of time without eating. As humans we are evolutionarily suited to endure intermittent fasts (16-24 hours) – original mankind (endogenous man) only ate when food was available, not continuously from a 24 hour vending machine.

Fasting is something you will learn to appreciate in a landscape of food abuse. Choosing not to eat may seem odd but it is clearly a path toward developing much better metabolic health.

Intermittent fasting and calorie restriction are directly linked to improving our insulin sensitivity. If we want to reduce harmful inflammation, oxidation and improve our body composition, utilize fat mass, and shed pounds then intermittent fasting (IF) is something we need to include in the components of our lifestyle.

Research indicates that **calorie restriction** and **intermittent fasting** are strongly linked to:

- **Slowing the Aging Process**
- **Promoting Metabolic Fitness and Health**

Research into intermittent fasting, uncovers a list of benefits and a simple truth that humans have been metabolically undergoing intermittent fasts for thousands of years.

Dynamics of Time Restricted Eating (TRE)

Intermittent fasting- that structures food intake around various activities and workouts is called Time Restricted Eating (TRE). The purpose is to develop a **FAT ADAPTED** metabolism providing an optimal environment for your mitochondria to **EXCEL** at the production of **ATP** whilst reducing increased Inflammation and Oxidation.

Our bodies are uniquely designed to transition smoothly between 'Fed' and Unfed, or 'Fasted' states.

In the fed state:

- Burning of fat is halted as insulin level is elevated. Insulin signals our body to store excess calories as fat cells, or stores of adiposity. In the presence of insulin, our body will burn glucose (from our last meal) instead of fat leaving access to our fat stores locked.

In the fasted state:

- Fat Storage is mobilized and our bodies start to utilize stored body fat (adiposity) as ATP energy substrate- instead of glucose.

While glucagon and growth hormone are elevated, insulin levels remain low. Our body starts mobilizing the substrate of body fat (adiposity) to create ATP and does so with far less ROS emission, and the cascade of inflammation and oxidation that the burning of sugar (carbohydrate) creates, it also yields- nearly 4-times as much energy- in the form of ATP energy.

NOTE: We best utilize stores of body fat (adiposity) while in a fasted (unfed) state, counter to our fed state, where we store body fat.

Societal Problems to Overcome

We are spending less and less of our time in a fasted (Unfed) state. Are we afraid we will starve? With this pattern, when does our poor metabolism ever get the chance to take out the metabolic trash (autophagy) and burn some fat?

- Our bodies and cells spend less and less time utilizing stored body fat for ATP energy. Our glycolic (sugar burning) pathways are being overused.
- The end result is insulin remains **high all the time** whilst our body becomes sugar dependent and avoids the burning of stored body fat. This reliance on Sugar is not unlike a heroin user's reliance on opioids.
- Don't be that over weight sugar zombie out there lugging all that fat around looking for "Energy"!
- Too much secretion of insulin leads to **'insulin resistance'** here the body secretes even more insulin in response to a fed state. **Obesity, abdominal fat storage, high triglycerides, low HDL** all contributes to **increased Inflammation** and **Oxidation (High CRP Levels).**

Isn't it about time we address the sobering reality of our state of health and make our goal to improve evidence based biomarkers, and worry less about how our butt looks in a swim suit?

The truth is when we get our markers in line, our butts will look great, and it is a positive side effect - unlike the list of nightmare side effects that stem from pharmaceutical use, food abuse, and fitness program abuse.

Sugar and Mitochondria

The mitochondria can burn either glucose (sugar) or fat for fuel, and over time they will have a preference for one over the other; **"sugar burners"** have increased the pathways into our mitochondria that burn glucose, and decreased, or down-regulated, the underused pathway for burning fat (fat utilization).

Fat and Mitochondria

Humans have the ability to become **'Fat Adapted'** and we improve our ability to fuel ourselves with stored body fat- instead of glucose. However, this takes time and practice, and our sugar abused body has to do a number of things to slowly up-regulate (or increase) our fat-burning pathways. Everything we do at **M360** will target our increased ability to become more, and more **FAT ADAPTED**!

Metabolic Benefits and the Wisdom of Fasting

Reducing total calorie intake is the only proven way to increase our lifespan.

Reduce calorie intake by 25%, and we can potentially add years to our life. Reducing our food intake is the only thing science has come up with that will increase our longevity and healthspan. Why not give it a try you may actually gain some healthspan, or just shed some fat mass in the process of trying.

Research also suggests that calorie restriction (CR) can delay the onset of many age-related diseases including:

- Heart disease
- Diabetes
- Hypertension
- Cancer

Multiple studies have discovered incredible benefits of CR and intermittent fasting, here are some of the benefits below:

- **Reduced hs CRP/Reduced inflammation**
- **Increased HDL cholesterol (the good cholesterol)**
- **Reduced triglycerides**
- **Reduced blood pressure**
- **Reduced cancer risk (tumor growth and progression)**
- **Increased fat utilization (Beta Oxidation of Excess Fat Mass)**
- **Improved body composition and Strength to weight Ratio**
- **Improved Insulin Sensitivity**

Intermittent fasting is an **incredibly powerful tool to normalize our glucose levels**. Moderate and measured exercise- in conjunction with intermittent fasting is one of the most powerful and natural insulin sensitizers we can adopt.

Effects of of intermittent fasting on metabolic diseases are listed here:

- **Increased insulin sensitivity**
- **Reduced post-prandial (after meal) blood glucose**
- **Reduced glucose variability (spike and diving)**
- **Reduced fasting blood glucose**

Intermittent fasting has been proven to improve insulin sensitivity

Intermittent Fasting (**IF**) enhances the utilization of fat in our liver and muscle tissue.

Insulin resistance promotes the accumulation fat tissue where it is not designed to be stored- in our muscle tissue and liver. Fatty Liver Disease (FLD) is an increasingly serious problem with today's youth.

When we restrict food intake for periods of time our bodies will have no choice but to utilize our stored fat (adiposity) as a prime substrate to create ATP energy. When we go without eating for short period of time, our fat stores are released (mobilized), and become powerful fuel our cells need to operate efficiently.

As lipid (fat) in our muscle and liver cells is reduced, our cells become increasingly responsive to insulin. When we reduce fat in our liver and muscle insulin becomes more powerful as a metabolic agent.

Oxidized LDL Deposits in Blood Vessels

The elasticity of our vasculature (Blood Vessels) is very important. The easier glucose and insulin can circulate in our bloodstream, and the easier they can cross blood vessel walls, the less high blood sugar levels we will have. Less oxidation and inflammation lends itself to normal blood vessels. **M360** targets the contents of our day, exercise, diet, and stress management to reduce oxidation and inflammation at every level of our life! **Why?**

1. With age and abuse fat (lipid) deposits can accumulate and oxidize LDL on the inside wall or blood vessel walls (endothelial wall).
2. Oxidized LDL's harden vessel walls and increase blood pressure- whilst increasing the potential to form blood clots- obstruct blood vessels- and ultimately lead to heart attack and stroke. HELLO wakeup call?

Calorie Restriction, Intermittent Fasting and TRE are vital to our Healthspan.

Studies indicate that time restricted eating (TRE); intermittent fasting (IF) and calorie restriction (CR), can reduce the negative vascular conditions of aging. Together these behaviors can:

- Reduce LDL cholesterol
- Increase HDL
- Reduce arterial blockage
- Reduce blood pressure
- Improve the transport of glucose and insulin across the vessel walls.

IF Changes the Function of Cells, Genes and Hormones

In the absence of food, several metabolic changes occur in our body. In the absence of food our bodies initiate important cellular repair processes (Autophagy) that mobilize stored body fat as a usable substrate for the metabolic creation of ATP.

A few of the changes that occur in our body during IF, CR and TRE are:

- **Fat Adaption/Utilization** which facilitates lower Insulin levels
- Higher levels of human growth hormone (HGH) along with increased fat utilization and muscle gain, along with other good metabolic events.
- Cells are repaired and waste removed senescent cells are removed and new growth is stimulated.
- Beneficial changes in **gene expression** related to longevity and protection against disease are increased.

>**BULLET POINT:** Insulin levels drop and human growth hormone increases when you fast.

Lose Weight and Belly Fat

Intermittent fasting by default will have you eating fewer meals and along with all the metabolic improvements you will lose weight specific to fat mass.

IF improves hormone function and facilitates weight loss while stimulating lean mass

Less insulin means higher growth levels of Human Growth Hormone (HGH). When HGH is increased norepinephrine (noradrenaline) is also increased stimulating the breakdown of body fat to be utilized as energy.

- **Fasting boosts your metabolic rate** (increases calories out)
- **Fasting reduces the volume or load of food you eat** (reduces calories in).

Research supports intermittent fasting as a tool to utilize 3-8% fat mass in just 5-8 weeks.

Intermittent fasting is an incredibly powerful FAT loss tool.

>**BULLET POINT:** Intermittent fasting is an effective tool to reduce fat mass- specifically belly fat- by boosting our metabolism in conjunction with TRE, moderate intensity exercise, and physical activity.

16-24 hours of fasting can Reduce Insulin Resistance

We must adopt methods and behaviors to lower our insulin resistance and be more insulin sensitive to protect ourselves against: inflammation and oxidation. Fasting is one such tool we should certainly adopt into our lifestyle.

Are you moving toward, or away from Oxidative Stress & Inflammation!

One of the single biggest steps we can take toward chronic disease is to increase our level of Oxidative Stress (OS). OS damages DNA with unpaired free radical ROS.

Once again- multiple studies link intermittent fasting as a very productive solution toward improving our metabolic defense against silent inflammation and Oxidative Stress (OS).

IF, CR and TRE provide Heart Health Benefits

The world's biggest killer of humankind is currently heart disease.

A simple manipulation of when we eat and how we mix fasting into our lifestyle can improve many risk factors associated with Heart Disease such as: lower blood pressure, higher HDL cholesterol, lower Insulin Resistance, lower blood triglycerides, lower inflammatory markers of hs-CRP and optimal blood sugar levels. Are we ringing some bells here?

IF, CR and TRE Promote the Cellular Repair Processes

Simple manipulation of what we eat, when we eat it- centered around various feel good physical activities and specific **M360** exercise will initiate a much needed cellular cleansing, cellular waste removal program known as autophagy, as well as refresh, renew, and repair our metabolism (mitochondrial function).

Autophagy cleans out broken and dysfunctional proteins that build up over time. Autophagy clears out dysfunctional- half life senescent cells. This clean up can protect us from a cascade of potential chronic diseases. I call these half life senescent cells, **"Thug Cells"** they just hang around and cause trouble, getting in the way of our good cells.

IF, CR and TRE can help in the Prevention of Cancer

Uncontrolled growth of cells is a horrible condition of Cancer. Again IF, CR and TRE have shown promising beneficial effects on our metabolism than reduce the risk of cancer.

Amongst cancer patients fasting showed to assist in the reduction of chemotherapy side effects.

IR, CR and TRE can benefit our Brain

Meal and lifestyle manipulation will benefit our brain by reducing OS and again, lowering our I-R Scores and even growing new nerve cells which is directly linked to benefit our brain function.

IR, CR and TRE have been associated with the stimulation of brain-derived neurotrophic factor –or- BDNF for short. Low levels of BDNF are associated with depression and other various brain issues.

Alzheimer's disease altered by IF, CR and TRE

Since there is no current cure for Neurodegenerative diseases like Alzheimer's and Parkinson's, preventing them from developing is critical. Research links Intermittent Fasting (IF), Calorie Restriction (CR), and Time Restricted Eating (TRE), along with- quality moderate intensity exercise, as a lifestyle intervention that shows preventative promise to reduce new cases.

Intermittent Fasting May Extend our Lifespan, Helping us Live Longer

Life and Healthspan extension is the most exciting effects of TRE, IF and CR.

Animal studies have demonstrated that test animals fed every other day lived 83% longer than those fed daily.

Want to live a longer and healthier life?

Given the known benefits of the various patterns of FASTING, to our metabolism and the improvement of so many health bio-markers, it makes sense to give it a try. I have been doing it for a few years now and it is simply amazing! I wake everyday with bounding energy and passion to spread this word to others. My experience is what has driven this book, podcast and M360 Clinical Fitness Center. I am **ON FIRE** with enthusiasm to help others (YOU)!

Why Not just Exercise More and Eat Less?

Being over-fat and obese is a very real epidemic. Being over-fat is a much bigger problem than just counting calories.

- Obesity is a metabolic condition!
- Obesity is a case of silent inflammation!
- Obesity disrupts healthy metabolic function!

To begin to reduce excessive fat we must disrupt the current signal within our hypothalamus that tells us to EAT!

1. The first step toward achieving this is to lower our level of silent inflammation.
2. The second step is not so much in reducing volume of food eaten, as it is altering the NUTRACEUTICAL CONTENT of what we eat and HOW OFTEN.
3. The end result is to alter our metabolism to become better FAT ADAPTED, yet satiated with a reduction of overall inflammation and OS.

Exercising more and eating less is an endless loop of misery and failure. We Must ALWAYS take our metabolism into account.

Ask yourself: How will my metabolism respond to what I am doing?

Anti-inflammatory Diets are a viable solution to our obesity epidemic

Anti-inflammatory diets that reduce silent inflammation make it easier to utilize fat and increase energy. Anti-inflammatory diets can also reduce and eliminate lipotoxicity and the cascade of chronic conditions leading to chronic disease.

How many more reasons do you need to finally understand the importance of become better fat adapted?

Metabolically Control body weight to Reduce Silent Inflammation

Let's gain metabolic control or our body composition by re-establishing our normal hormone balance that will satisfy our metabolism with satiety instead of the growling hunger of too much hunger hormone (ghrelin).

Manipulating our metabolism to reduce silent inflammation induced by poor lifestyle choices should be our starting point. We must be able to formulate an anti-inflammatory diet based on Nutraceutical value that can be used like a Pharmaceutical- administered at the right time to effectively reduce and control silent inflammation.

hs -CRP (C - reactive protein) is the Key Biomarker of Inflammation

More and more evidence is coming in that inflammation and oxidation of LDL contributes to atherogenesis. hs-**C-reactive protein** (hs CRP) levels can finally bring us into the light and reflect for us the critical level of overall total body inflammation levels.

Remember: Show me inflammation and oxidation and I will show you chronic conditions that can lead to chronic disease.

The scale for your high sensitivity – C Reactive Protein (hs-CRP) blood test is here:

Score and Risk for Future Cardiovascular event:

- **Low Risk- less than <1.00 mg/L**
- **Average Risk – 1.00 – 3.00 mg/L**
- **High Risk > 3.00 mg/L**

It is my opinion that everyone should have this inexpensive test done, to confirm your current level of Inflammation- relative to the chosen components of your lifestyle.

HOW inflamed are you? _____

A HIGH LEVEL of **CRP** in the blood is a marker of high silent inflammation.

Question: If you had high CRP levels and documented high levels of Silent Inflammation that cause all these horrible chronic diseases, wouldn't it make sense to initiate a Nutraceutical Intervention complete with evidence based, feel good exercise and physical activity to reduce inflammation and achieve wellness and better human performance?

YES of Course you may respond!

Then **WHY** in most cases are the above situations treated with even more inflammation causing- pharmaceuticals with dangerous side effects and interactions?

Isn't the goal as **Dr. Mark Potzler** so gracefully stated- to improve health and reduce pharmaceutical dependency?

The key to our **M360** program is to reduce your total body inflammation within the first 5-week block of our "**all inclusive**"- intervention program. Your health and human performance is based on identifying lifestyle behaviors, routines and activities that will start reducing your overall – Measurable State of Inflammation. **Together we can do this!**

Lower CRP by targeting: Lifestyle, Diet, Exercise & Stress Mgmt.

Can we lower your CRP? Will lower CRP reduce detrimental health risk? There's no doubt that the very best way to lower CRP is through:

- **Lifestyle Makeover**
- **Physical Activity/Exercise**
- **Diet/Nutrition**
- **Stress/Recovery**

The power of optimizing your lifestyle extends beyond just CRP. Studies show in addition to lower CRP levels:

- **Lipid ratios came down**
- **Insulin levels came down**

These processes are all interlinked and changeable by our behavior and choice of lifestyle.

Studies the anti-inflammatory benefits of moderate exercise are independent of weight loss with studies showing that CRPs fell whether or not the patients lost weight. Sure it is nice to lose fat weight, if your composition is that of too much body fat as a percentage of total weight, but the health benefits of M360 exercise comes first. Being lean and beautiful is a side effect of being metabolically efficient and healthy. This is our focus at **M360**.

We will of course go into further detail in later sections of this book, how to specifically address biomarkers of inflammation and oxidation. Summary of steps are:

- Upgrade your lifestyle as we are discussing to include new effective components
- Include appropriate moderate exercise that activates & promotes the power of our ANS recovery phase

- Modify our diet- Cut out sugar, additives, refined grains, starches and processed food in general.
- Consume more Omega 3, more nuts, fish, avocado, olive oil.
- More foods rich in antioxidants like berries and vegetables that are brightly colored.
- Add in Vitamin C, E and Omega 3 supplements
- Reduce Stress by becoming better aware of what triggers stress. Better sleep and learning to exhale.

What makes our program different is we are not just focusing on vanity and the weight scale, we are focusing on:

- **MEASURABLE**
- **DOCUMENTABLE**

CLINICAL FITNESS!

- **Health Longevity**
- **Anti Aging**
- **Higher Human Performance**

We can live a healthier life, full of joy and fruitful activity while eating foods and enjoying moderate exercise routines that promote Anti-Inflammation and Anti- Oxidation the precious cells of our body and state of our mind.

You can execute these programs at a certified metafit.life **M360** facility near you. For more information go to: **www.metafit.life** and listen to our podcast: **Power 2 Learn** on iTunes, Google Play and Podbean.

Wouldn't it make sense to document the inflammatory state of a patient's metabolism and prescribe a lifestyle, diet, exercise and relaxation program to lower the state of inflammation and reduce or eliminate symptoms of Chronic Disease?

Are you that patient? Yes/No

If you do not change some components of your lifestyle, will you be that patient? Yes/No_____

Dynamics of Sleep and Inflammation:

Keep in mind the most important part of our 24hr day is **SLEEP!** Recovery is the key theme of this book! WE cannot have effective recovery without proper **SLEEP!**

Recovery, as you will see – manifests itself in every section of this book.

Without RECOVERY we have NOTHING!

Without RECOVERY we are Metabolically Bankrupt!

- **How do you sleep?** _____
- **What do you consider a good night's sleep?**_____
- **Are you set up for successful deep sleep?** _____

Sleep affects a cascade of events that promote or sabotage our metabolic function. Poor sleep increases appetite by reducing Leptin which drives our hunger for more high carbohydrate foods. When you get to section 3 this will make a lot more sense.

Do you have cravings for carbohydrates and sweets?

Sleep is strongly linked to metabolic processes that are critical to maintain our metabolic/hormonal balance. The entire theme- in fact the **TITLE** of this book is: **Metabolic Fitness for LIFE!** You cannot have optimal metabolic health without proper sleep and recovery.

Sleep deprivation creates a much bigger issue of circadian misalignment that wreaks chaos on our metabolism through a variety of ways causing:

hormonal imbalance, sympathetic overstimulation, and you guessed it: **INFLAMMATION**.

Take note on the overstimulation of your sympathetic nervous system as we will be discussing **Heart Rate Variability (HRV)** measurement as one of your tools to monitor and regulate detrimental overstimulation of our stress response.

Our metabolism is the entire range of biochemical processes that occur within our body as a living organism.

We now know our metabolism is comprised of two distinct metabolic processes:

1. **Anabolism** (build up)
2. **Catabolism** (break down)

Our Metabolism- in general- is associated with cellular injury due to the release of free radicals/ROS (Reactive Oxygen Species), as a byproduct of our metabolism, in particular- our sugar metabolism. Sleep is the key to defending our body against the negative effects of Free Radical Damage. Both anabolism and catabolism are important, and SLEEP is what negotiates the balance between these two powerful metabolic pathways.

HOW well do you currently balance Anabolism and Catabolism?

Proper sleep will <u>LOWER</u> our Metabolic Rate and Brain Temperature- allowing our body the opportunity to- address catabolic damage done to our cells - during waking hours.

Sleep and Recovery is Critical to your Metabolic Health!

Metabolic health and Sleep/Recovery is critical for us to understand. Without proper sleep and recovery from life and exercise our entire thesis of **Optimal Health** goes down the drain!!!! Our buzz words are

RECOVERY and **Feel Good** physical activities that enrich and fulfill your **Lifestyle.** It is incredibly important to us that you **FEEL GOOD!**

Glucose Regulation, Growth Hormone and Cortisol Levels

Growth hormone and cortisol, as you know -are two hormones that have an impact on our glucose regulation.

Our **M360** exercise and nutritional philosophy is to improve our metabolic health and performance to achieve sustainable metabolic fitness for life. As we should all agree by now, the most important part of any 24 hour cycle is our 8 hour sleep cycle.

Cortisol and growth hormone (HGH) are very active during various levels of sleep. Cortisol is most active during REM sleep and Growth Hormone is elevated during slow wave sleep (SWS) at the beginning, or onset of sleep. I hope you will start to see how our entire 30,000 foot view/Global perspective of health and performance depends on optimal sleep recovery.

Poor sleep, or lack of sleep can damage our immune response and increase pro-inflammatory markers as reflected in our: High Sensitivity – C Reactive Protein levels (hs-CRP). In addition to increasing inflammation and free radical oxidation, sleep deprivation can result in reduced glucose tolerance.

Introduction to Inflammation and Cardio death

The connection between inflammation and atherosclerosis has been around since the 19th century. As I write this book and review the studies it makes so much common sense. Inflammation brings with it oxidation, and it becomes quite clear that oxidized LDL's damage and injure our endothelium or blood vessel walls. With this damage, oxidation and excess of ROS (reactive oxygen species) it is a perfect environment for plaque buildup, much like a scab, **NOW** you are in trouble as there is now an opportunity for blockage and with it strokes and heart attacks.

The connection between chronic inflammation and has prompted effective ways to detect silent inflammation. The current gold standard of silent inflammation detection is: high sensitivity (hs) C-reactive protein (hs-CRP) as a biomarker of inflammation, leading to oxidation and a window to potential blood vessel damage.

Let me ask you this: If you were at a fork in the road, and you knew that a right turn meant agonizing death- while a left turn meant safety and a smooth ride home, which turn would you pick, right or left?

Why not get our hs-CRP checked and with it take a swing at the content of this book and change a few things in our life before it is too late?

- When you look behind the curtain of cardiovascular disease you quickly find a variety of conditions that are detrimentally affected by Inflammation:
  ○ Insulin resistance
  ○ Visceral obesity
  ○ Metabolic syndrome and type 2- diabetes

You guessed it: Conditions of Inflammation and Oxidation are once again revealed!

- Cardiovascular risk has long been associated with physical inactivity. Studies are quite clear on how proper **"Moderate & Measured"** physical activity can raise mood and improve nitric oxide pathways, whilst improving vasodilatation and the stimulation of endogenous, anti-inflammatory mechanisms.

Five biomarkers we can control for the elimination of Chronic Disease are:

(1) Chronic Inflammation and Free Radical Oxidation (ROS)
(2) Heart Rate Variability (HRV)
(3) Post Exercise Recovery Rate (PERR)
(4) Strength to Weight Ratio (STWR)
(5) Mobility, Balance & Flexibility (Biomechanics of Movement)

The thesis of our book, podcast and program are to take on:

- **10- Critical Biomarkers** of our health over a:
- **8-12-week "Block"** of our life, in:
- **15-modalities** along with
- **Daily Learning** (Power 2 Learn Podcast) to dramatically improve your
- **Personal knowledge to SUSTAIN a NEW**
- **HEALTHY - PERFORMANCE BASED** behaviors and routines.

WE must develop and arm ourselves with new structures of life- to formulate a winning lifestyle -that will optimize our health span, and reduce morbidity.

As you can see it all starts and ends with SLEEP!

Without proper sleep the benefits of the other 3- sections of this book, are **VOID**!

A comment you will hear quite often in my writings is:

"WE must change our direction -to change our outcome, so knowing where we are, and where we are going, is critical to the success of our program" tb

For this reason I hope you feel like we are having a conversation as you read my writing.

How do you sleep?

The words **METABOLISM** and **LIFE** are the same to me. **Life** comes from the process of your **Metabolism** and specifically the function of your **Mitochondria**. I want this book to be simple. You need not have a degree in Biochemistry to understand it. For this reason I will speak in over simplistic terms.

HOW does your Lifestyle - Sleep and Recovery - affect the efficiency of your - Mitochondrial Health?

Pace of Aging

All of us are aging, time is ticking, and the question is NOT "Are you Aging", but rather at what **PACE** are you aging?

- We all age at a different pace.
- What controls the pace, genetics or lifestyle, or both, and how much control do we have? More than you think and it is time to exercise your control!
- What can you start doing today to affect your pace of aging?

Immortality

Aging is the common denominator of all human beings. No one person is getting younger that I am aware of? Many of the studies I have read state the every changing structure and nature of Metabolic Function and theories of aging. Most researchers are finding that lifespan and healthspan can be dramatically extended with the adoption of simple choices we can all make. Choices like IF intermittent fasting, CR calorie restriction and TRE time restricted eating. Our modern society rarely goes any substantial time without eating.

Listen to some of the research from USC professor via Podcast by **Dr. Valter Longo**; I think you will be amazed at how simple improving our health may be.

What science in finding is that when we go periods without food our body simply has an opportunity to repair itself? As crazy as it may sound there are more and more conversations including the topic of Immortality!

Longevity and Healthspan

With $2.9 trillion of $3.2 trillion in total healthcare being spent on **Chronic Disease** it is quite clear we **CANNOT** continue on this path! As we age and these diseases start showing up- with no cure- these age associated diseases become the greatest challenges and financial burdens the United States has ever faced. **What are we doing about it?**

- The sad state of our existence is the fact that over the last 100 years our longevity has grown, but **NOT** our Healthspan. We have far too many aging chronically sick people sitting around lonely and not really enjoying this existence. It makes me sad and at the same time it pisses me off. Have you ever looked into a few medicine cabinets of people 85-95 years of age? I know because my own mother is 87 as of this writing. I see it every day where she lives, and in and out of the ER, and doctor's offices. Are you going to clean up your act **NOW** and start utilizing some of the Metabolic Interventions I am making you aware of, or are you going to continue on the path you are on, one that common census tells us- is a path of ever and ever increasing Inflammation and Oxidation from poor lifestyle, physical activity, diet and stress mgmt. choices. Uninformed choices that do not have to be made.

Aging Biomarkers are defined as:

- **Metabolic Characteristics that can be measured objectively with evidence based biomarkers as we age.**

The following is a list of biomarkers **M360** will simplify. Why not put some effort- as a society, into indentifying and improving biomarkers that decrease our healthspan? Here are some anti-aging targets **M360** will track:

1. **Standards Measurements of Power- Vitality and Function (PVF)**
   A. As we age we **DO NOT** want to become **FRAIL!**
   B. Our **M360 goal** is to immediately arrest the slide of:
      1. Strength
      2. Endurance, and-
      3. Physical Ability along with…
      4. Cognitive Function!

Left **UN-ARRESTED** these states will leave you vulnerability to more and more: Chronic Disease – Dependence and Death!

   C. We will look at **Power** at the Athletic Champion Level
   D. We will look at **Vitality** at the everyday Recreational Level
   E. We will look at **Function** and increasing healthspan.

At what point in our lives do we make that dramatic metabolic shift from **YOUNG** to **OLD?**

It seems our society is split in philosophy with attitudes of:

"Oh you are too <u>YOUNG</u> to worry about behavior interventions to your Lifestyle, Physical Activity, Diet and Stress Mgmt.

<OR>

Oh you are too <u>OLD</u> to change, alter or biohack your markers of health, performance and longevity.

Starting **TODAY**, regardless of your age you must take it upon yourself to know and take interest in the markers of your own **HEALTH** and **PERFORMANCE! Bio-Markers you should be Interested in:**

- Insulin Resistance
- Insulin Response to personal foods
- DEXA (abdominal adiposity)
- HDL
- Triglycerides
- Blood pressure
- Inflammatory markers (hs-CRP)
- Epigenetic profile
- PERR Post Exercise Recovery Rate
- 6 minute recovery rate (yo/yo)
- Strength and Mobility reference points
- Strength to Wt ratio's

Aging, Chronic Disease and Human Choice all go hand in hand

Research evidence suggests that targeting aging can- not only postpone chronic diseases, but also prevent a variety of debilitating age-associated metabolic conditions whilst extending our healthy lifespan.

Metafit.life M360's goal is to identify, educate, and change health outcomes simply by becoming aware of the metabolic issues such as Oxidation and the variety of lifestyle intervention we can all employ today with great opportunity to dramatically increase our quality healthspan and reduce morbidity.

M360 is all about more of us recognizing the following metabolic pathways of:

- Anabolism
- Catabolism
- Inflammation
- Oxidation
- Epigenetic modifications that can alter our rate of aging and proclivity toward age-related chronic disease

WE can <u>BIOHACK</u> our health- and <u>ALTER</u> outcomes <u>TODAY!</u>

Lifestyle modifications -Nutraceutical adaptations, and Moderate/Measured **FEEL GOOD** Exercise, along with NEW stress release techniques can change our life forever! All of these Interventions are relatively simple and can be started today! What are you waiting for?

Immediate Interventions that will start changing your health NOW!

These include:

1. **Intermittent Fasting** (IF)
2. **Time Restricted Eating** (TRE)
3. **Calorie Reduction** (CR)
4. **Free Fatty Acid Aerobic Training** (FFA)
5. **Aerobic Transition Point Training** (ATP)
6. **Sub Lactate Threshold "Higher Intensity" Training** (LT HIIT)
7. **50/70 RPT resistance training (50/70)**
8. **Low glycemic diet, protein timing and dietary fat balance**
9. **Epigenetics**
10. **Proper Sleep and Recovery (ability to relax on the fly)**

We may have more control over our _Genetic Outcomes_ than you think!

What does that mean?

Here is a crash course in biochemistry and genetics:

- The working units of every human being are the cells of our body. Our DNA holds all the instructions that are required for our bodies to constantly renew ourselves at the cellular level.
- Our **Genes** provide instructions on how to make important building block proteins – and trigger a variety of biological actions that renew and regenerate new life within us from the old –or– become sick and die. **We have control of our health and performance outcomes**

I have heard expressions like this over my lifetime as a facilitator:

- **"I am fat because I am big boned"** or
- **"Oh, heart disease runs in my family"**, is this true?

I have even heard:

- **"I cannot reduce my carbohydrate consumption because I am Italian and we eat lotsa pasta"** or
- "**I cannot reduce my carbohydrate consumption of white tortillas, because I am Hispanic"**, is this true?

Is any of this true, or are these convenient excuses?

Heart disease may be a genetic proclivity, but flour tortillas are **NOT**! We may have more control of our genetics as a result of a term known as epigenetic.

What is Epigentics?

Think of two different classrooms, same subject, same books/learning tools, and two different teachers.

- Think of your **lifespan** as the duration of these two classes.
- Think of the **cells** of our body as the students of these two classrooms.

- Think of your **DNA** as the syllabus or script of activity assigned to each class.
- Think of your **genetics** as the content of the script or syllabus, the actual words and topics.
- Think of Epigentics as the Director or Teacher/Facilitator/ Leader of content. (YOU)
- The facilitator is **YOU**, how you **CHOOSE** to express your Lifestyle similar to your genetic expression.

The classrooms, students and course content can be the same, but the expression can be totally different.

How we write our Lifestyle, choose and execute various simple components dictate outcomes or expressions of our life. In other words we can alter the EXPRESSION of our Genes.

What do you choose, and how do you express it? It is up to YOU!

This is what this book is all about.

You do **NOT** have to be fat because you are Italian and you do **NOT** have to die of heart disease because your dad did!

You have the **POWER** to modify and tweak your genetic expressions and health outcomes, healthspan and performance level!

Epigenetics is the study of changes in organisms- caused by *modification of gene expression*- rather than alteration of the genetic code itself.

Epigenetics and Chronic Disease

Most- if not all Chronic Disease results from the interaction between genetic predisposition and external factors, such as diet, exercise, stress, smoking, environmental exposure and loneliness. Notice loneliness, sometimes a simple pet like a dog can change your life. Maybe Dog's really are man's best friend? Mine sure is.

Epigenetic Harmony and Chosen Lifestyle Factors

In conclusion to this first section, the term lifestyle is broadly used to describe the **"typical way of life or manner of living characteristic of an individual or group"**. This concept includes different factors such as diet, behavior, stress, physical activity, working habits, smoking and alcohol consumption. Individual genetic background and environmental factors are intertwined to lifestyle in determining the health status of individuals.

Just as the conductor of an orchestra controls the dynamics of a symphonic performance, epigenetic factors govern the interpretation of DNA within each living cell. It all truly comes down the health and environment of your life as an organism at the cellular level. Metabolic Fitness for Life is a controllable equation you must act on.

Everything at **M360** points at reducing Inflammation and Oxidation to provide a Measurable Cascade of Positive Health Improvements.

Bio Marker Information relative to M360 inspired lifestyle

The following **Clinical Biomarkers** of NMR testing and Exercise Test is what we will hold our **M360 Metabolic Fitness for Life Program** accountable to:

Bio Markers M360 will Target:	*My Own as of 7/22/2018*	Health Standard	YOU?
1. hs CRP (High > Lower)	**.43**	<1.5 m/L	_____
2. Triglycerides (High > Lower)	**53** mg/dL	<150 mg/dL	_____
3. HDL (Low >Higher)	**87** mg/dL	>40 mg/dL	_____
4. Insulin Scale (**IR Score** Resistant → Sensitive)	**<25** (0-100)	<45 (0-100)	_____
5. Blood Pressure (High >Lower)	**110/65** mmHg	< 120/80mmHg	
6. Lean Mass/Fat Mass (LM/FM)	**90.5%/9.5%**	80%/20%	

7. Post Exercise Recovery Rate (1 and 2 Minute Recovery/ Max/ Sub max

8. Strength to Weight Ratio 250 watts 20 minutes @80% vs 200 watts @ 70%

9. Resting Heart Rates and HRV (Activation and De Activation of ANS)

10. Mobility, Balance & Range of Motion (ROM)

Sections 2-3-4 will pinpoint:

- Physical Activity/Exercise
- Diet/Nutrition
- Stress Management/Relaxation

Keep in mind this book is not a **NOVEL**, it is a reference guide to our **M360** program. **M360** is a clinical approach to achieving **Metabolic Fitness for Life** by arming patient/clients with the tools they need to put us **OUT** of **BUSINESS!**

Section #1 Summary:

Sleep is the most important component of our 24 hour day. The first goal of any program we embark upon should be to optimize this special 8 hour period of sleep/recovery for optimal metabolic health. **Who here is going to argue that?**

This leaves 16 hours each day for us to shape into a winning formula. What are you and I going to do with it? **This is our Lifestyle!**

We know what is killing us- we know that **Inflammation** leads to **Oxidative Stress**- which leads to the silent brewing of chronic conditions- that ultimately rear their ugly heads as **Chronic Disease**. We can now measure inflammation with a simple inexpensive blood test called an hs-CRP. **What is your CRP?**

We know that the total bill for US Healthcare at last CDC check- was $3.2 Trillion Dollars, of which a whopping $2.9 Trillion Dollars of that is spent on Chronic Disease!

Chronic Disease by definition is neither a condition we can vaccinate against, nor is it a condition we can treat with pharmaceuticals. Chronic Disease is, for the most part, a product of making consistently bad lifestyle decisions.

Am I silly to think that we who read this material and become aware of a few absolute metabolic truths, in a landscape of deceit and abuse- would not benefit from learning?

We simply do not know- what we do not know, but we can change it!

Take time to re-read this section and write down a few things you can adopt into your 16 hours, do your own research and you will see we have a **LOT MORE POWER** than you may realize. We can modify and optimize our metabolism with a variety of modalities we **"CHOOSE"** to execute.

When you find a sustainable schedule and start to work your own personal "winning" variety of components, and you start to see and feel the metabolic change- then it is our duty to **SHARE** it with a friend. This is how we get better as a society.

SECTION #2

Exercise

Physical Activities

LIFESTYLE COMPONENT #2

Physical Activity/Exercise

The words **Physical Activity and Exercise** - just like the words diet and nutrition have been abused. All the misinformation we are bombarded with totally confuses the real biomarkers and methods of proper-physical activity and exercise to achieve our **M360** objective of:

Metabolic Fitness for Life

While people may be getting better at rolling a tire around a room, they are certainly not getting anymore metabolically fit and healthy.

Is your Fitness Program <u>FAILING</u> to improve your Health?

The words **"Fit"** and **"Healthy"** are often used harmoniously in our language; yet the terms have entirely different meanings.

- Fitness describes the ability to perform a specific exercise task
- Health explains a person's measurable state of well-being, where physiological systems work in harmony (CRP, HDL, BP, Triglycerides, and Insulin Sensitivity).

We may view athletes as fit and healthy, yet oftentimes they simply-
ARE NOT!

The global term we place on unhealthy athletes is Overly Oxidized and Inflamed- Overtraining Syndrome. **M360** suggests a few primary drivers contributing to the development of unhealthy fitness programs and people who take part in them are:

- **Too Much High Intensity Interval Training (Metabolic Acidosis)**
- **Highly processed, high glycemic diet (Simple Carbohydrates)**
- **Poor Fat adaption (FAT Oxidation Capacity)**
- **Poor Aerobic Capacity- (Sub Maximum Utilization of Oxygen)**

These factors elicit a **sympathetic nervous system** response driving systemic reactive oxygen species (ROS) production, inflammation, and a metabolic substrate imbalance:

- Activities and Exercises that drive our **Energy Metabolism TOWARD** Carbohydrate Utilization and **AWAY** from Fat Oxidation actually enhance chronic conditions- that lead to chronic disease.
- These activities and exercise regimes need to be identified and removed from your list of lifestyle components within your 16 hour day.

At the end of the day, these activities and conditions produce unhealthy people. **M360** would like to suggest that scientists, athletes and healthcare practitioners get on the **SAME PAGE** and start working together- toward optimal health, and reduce overtraining syndrome by:

- Lowering training intensity and educating clients to proper clinical exercise to achieve evidence based clinical fitness that is driven by the stimulation of our Fat Metabolism.

- Learn the value of said **FAT ADAPTION** and remove high glycemic/processed foods from our diet, which together would increase fat oxidation rates and lower free radical ROS.

Our Clinical Baseline Objective is to Become Better Fat Adapted!

M360: Athletes & Fitness Enthusiast should be **FIT** and **HEALTHY**.

How does M360 Clinical Fitness lead to improved health outcomes?

Multiple biological mechanisms are responsible for a reduced risk of chronic conditions that lead to chronic disease and premature death.

Quality physical activities and exercise routines have been shown to improve:

- Body composition (e.g., through reduced abdominal adiposity and improved weight control)
- Reduced triglyceride levels,
- Increased high-density lipoprotein [HDL]
- Improve glucose homeostasis and insulin sensitivity
- Reduce blood pressure
- Improve autonomic tone
- Reduce systemic inflammation
- Improve coronary blood flow
- Enhance endothelial function
- Reduce Chronic inflammation, as indicated by elevated circulating levels of inflammatory mediators such as C-reactive protein, has been shown to be strongly associated with most of the chronic diseases whose prevention has benefited from proper moderate exercise.

Recent Studies have shown that exercise training may cause marked reductions in C-reactive protein (CRP) levels. Each of these factors may explain directly or indirectly the reduced incidence of chronic disease and premature death among people who engage in proper evidence based exercise routines and physical activities that target- the improvement of specific- measurable human biomarkers noted above, and throughout this book.

We Must Change our Definitions to Better Affect Known Biomarkers

Here is our definition of Exercise and Physical Activity for the purpose of our **M360** program:

Definition of Physical Exercise is a specific physical activity that directly enhances or maintains measurable- metabolic health, wellness and human performance.

Exercise and Physical Activities are performed for various reasons including:

- **Power, Vitality, Function**
- **Endurance stamina**
- **Metabolic Fat Utilization**
- **Aerobic Capacity**
- **Composition alteration Fat Mass/Lean Mass**
- **Just plain enjoyment.**

NIH on Physical Activity and Exercise:

Physical activity is any body movement that works your muscles and requires more energy than resting. Walking, running, paddling, cycling, swimming, yoga, and gardening are a few examples of physical activity.

According to the Department of Health and Human Services, Physical Activity refers to movement that enhances health. Does your program enhance your health, if so what aspects, which biomarkers are you affecting and to what degree? Do you know?

- Optimize Blood Pressure
- Optimize Resting HRV
- Lower CRP
- Increase HDL
- Lower Triglyceride Levels
- Lower Excess Body Fat Mass
- Increase/Maintain Lean Mass
- Improve Strength to Weight Ratio
- Lower Insulin Resistance
- Lower Resting Heart Rate
- Improve Fat Metabolism (Fat Adapted)
- Lower Oxidative Stress
- Lower Inflammation
- Improve 1 and 2 minute active Post Max/Sub Max Recovery Rates
- Lower overall Stress and Improve Sleep depth/pattern
- Improve Respiration Resting and Threshold Breathing
- Improve Flexibility/Mobility/Suppleness
- Improve Mental Outlook and Motivation to Thrive

Regardless of whether you call what you choose to do: **"physical activity"** or **"physical exercise"**- people who engage in either –or- both have:

- **Lower inflammatory markers**
- **Lower Cardiovascular risk**

Our **KEY TARGET** at **M360** is the fact that studies have shown beneficial effects of properly done physical activity and exercise on reducing inflammation and oxidation markers.

Specific physical activity is referred to as exercise. Specific resistance training, specific aerobic or anaerobic training sessions, such as circuit training, cycling classes are examples of exercise. **M360** targets specific metabolic response, with specific evidence based exercise that is documentable. Each session is recorded and shared with you via email, text, Garmin Connect, and Strava immediately after your session.

Physical activity is good for many parts of your body. Physical activity is just one part of our heart-healthy **M360** lifestyle. A heart-healthy lifestyle also involves following a heart-healthy eating, aiming for a healthy weight, managing stress, and quitting smoking along with other bad habits and making better **Lifestyle Component Choices.**

M360 Physical Activities Target "Feel Good" Exercise

We live in a world of extremes. In a nutshell we humans do two things very well:

1. **Nothing**
2. **Too Much**

The major impetus for starting **M360** is a gaping **NEED** in our society to:

1. **Utilize science and technology to**
2. **Better target health and human performance**

A lot of what is going on in terms of commercial exercise programs is far too stressful on the human mind and body. The key successful program over the years is the ability to:

- **LOAD** and **RECOVER**
- **STIMULATE** and **IMPROVE**

I learned this at the Olympic Training Center from Leslie Shooter. She got me thinking about this very simple statement:

"Tim- it is all about loading and recovering. The trick is How Much to Load, How often, and getting the proper amount of recovery before you load again".

Dr. Vigil refers to it as the **Super Compensation Model**.

- Exercise breaks us down from our activity (Load) or metabolic state of *Catabolism*
- Recovery (Rest) builds us back up, in a metabolic state of *Anabolism* to a point slightly above where we started before previous training.

Done correctly proper training is a stair like progress into improved human performance at all levels. Done incorrectly as most programs and you destroy rather than stimulate the very metabolic process we seek to improve for long term health and sustainable performance.

Technology allows us to pinpoint the cornerstones of any physical activity:

1. **Intensity**
2. **Duration**
3. **Frequency**

Physical Activities should be as vigilant about:

- **Releasing, relaxing and recovering (Parasympathetic Activation), as they are about activating and recruiting muscle contraction (Sympathetic Activation).**

Make no mistake about it, when we refer to *"Feel Good"* exercise we mean it. There must be plenty of time allotted for recovery from intensities that *"Stimulate"* optimal cellular health versus - **too much intensity all the time** which degrades and damages cellular function. Are you listening Gym Rat's and Xfitters?

M360 targets the simple principles of *"Load and Recover"* and our aim is to document it with proof via blood test and measurable performance test like:

- Post Exercise Recover Rate (PERR)
- hs-CRP blood tests

Exercise and Physical Activities should *FEEL GOOD*, again -our process targets **STIMULATION** and Targets Evidence Based Exercise that takes the guesswork out of our efforts and investments into exercise and physical activity.

Pain, Pain, Go Away

Metafit Life 360's full circle approach is to help people to incorporate simple components of lifestyle to reduce Oxidation, Inflammation, to Optimize Health and Performance, whilst eliminating chronic conditions and chronic disease. This is our goal regardless of your physical state of being. From Olympic Athlete to a patient recovering from a heart attack, intensity, duration and frequency are relative to the patient's current state of being.

What the Research Shows

Think about your day? You wake up in a given state of mind and sense of well being, good, bad or ugly and you set out to face the next 16 hours of your life. How much pain and stress will you be put through today, at work, from life that comes at you, life that is out of your control, and then how much exercise or physical activity are you willing to put yourself through?

What do the cells of our body need?

How much time will you spend learning new ways to eat, such as functional eating, or how to best balance all aspects of life as well as- load and recover exercise, utilizing technology such as heart rate monitors, blood glucose monitors, HRV tracking devices, blood pressure monitors, specific blood test, recovery test?

You must- Assign Power and Sustainability to your Program

Research shows that those who assess and assign power to their program, and become involved in evidence based lifestyle programs, are far more capable of achieving and sustaining much better health and performance. The primary reason is they are executing **Meaningful Modalities** of evidence based activities while **LEARNING**.

Learning is the Key to Success!

Learning is invigorating, mind expanding and stimulates interest to solidify intrinsic motivation. Our ***Power 2 Learn Podcast*** was developed to assist you in learning simply by putting topics on the air for you to explore and choose your own level of knowledge. Find us on **iTunes** or **Google Play**, they are 100% Free.

Any person wanting to improve their health is going to be faced with a **self observed analysis of their own lifestyle** and part of any program to help you will advise real evidence based physical activity and exercise.

$2.9 Trillion Dollar Question:

Wouldn't it be best to take a few minutes before you engage in a program or activity- to better understand how your body works, and pinpoint the meaningful components of physical activity and exercise that drive metabolic need?

- **What are we doing and why?**
- **What is the short and long term effect?**
- **How sustainable is it?**
- **What Biomarkers does it affect and to what extent?**
- **How does it affect the course of my day, my life?**

Muscle Stress and Contraction Dynamics

When the body is stressed, muscles tense up. Muscle tension is a reaction to stress — a conditioned response to guard against injury and pain.

With sudden onset of stress, muscles tense up (concentric contraction) all at once, and then release their tension (eccentric contraction) when the stress passes, sometimes you will hold tension (isometric contraction) before releasing.

- **Concentric Contractions**
- **Eccentric Contractions**
- **Isometric Contractions**

These three **PHASES of MUSCULAR CONTRACTION** are the cornerstones of all movement- from walking to lifting a weight. Our goal is not so much about **WHAT** you do, as **HOW** you do it. How you feel it, and creating ways of making you want to repeat the movement. **Hence: A Feel Good Program!**

Chronic stress can create a state of constant of guardedness or low-grade contraction. Muscles that are tense for a long time may trigger other reactions of our body thus promoting a variety of stress disorders. We need to learn the metabolic value of relaxing and letting go of low level chronic contractions.

We take specific care to address this; our goal with everything in the **M360** program is to Feel Good, by paying attention to Tension, Stress and Perceived Pain. **Every aspect or component of our program is to:**

1. **Reduce Pain**
2. **Reduce Inflammation**
3. **Reduce Oxidation**
4. **Expand Aerobic Capacity**
5. **Improve Strength to Weight Ratio**
6. **Lower Fat Mass**
7. **Promote Metabolic Health & Fat Adaption**
8. **Improve HRV and Parasympathetic Activation**
9. **Improve Ability to Relax and Recover**
10. **Optimize Sleep and Stress Management**

Overtraining and the Hype of Fitness in Modern Society

Overtraining is a real danger if you work out every single day or more than once a day, if you have to make yourself exercise despite feeling wiped out, and if you do cardio or sprint workouts too often while only focusing on burning calories. There's a sweet spot for everyone, and it's up to you to monitor, track and discover what the proper amount is for you, work in partnership with your body — this way the right amount of exercise will comes naturally.

Personally I have a variety of activities that I teach and engage in, from Olympic K-1 paddling, 50/70 resistance sessions to indoor Zwift cycling competitions and training regiments- to leisurely Lap Swimming, Walking, Hiking, Yoga/Stretching, and Easy Mountain Bike Rides and Beach Cruiser Outings with my wife or stimulating 100 mile rides on my Road Bike. If I see my HRV is high upon waking and I feel tired, I may shift from the plan to do a heavy weight training session (70% 1rmax) and go for a 4 mile walk, or a session of lap swimming and Yoga. Be Flexible and keep it **FUN**. Learn how to **ADJUST** the **STRESS** knob **DOWN** as well as **UP!**

Too Much Stress = Chronic Response

Excessive sessions and blocks of exercise (load) paired with inadequate rest (recovery) and improper nutrition will result in acute inflammation that cascades into a chronic response, and with it injury, illness and burnout.

A recent paper I read presented overtraining as exercise-induced connective tissue and muscle trauma that triggers the release of ***pro-inflammatory cytokines.*** This is acute inflammation that results from excessive exercise with inadequate rest becoming a ***chronic response*** cascading into a systemic immune response that detrimentally involves the central nervous system (CNS), immune system, and liver.

Note: What is a Cytokine?

Short Answer: a Cytokine is a protein that is secreted by cells in many forms. They can come as Anti or Pro Inflammatory. We can really take you off in the weeds here, but the important thing to understand is that these little agents of health or destruction are a reaction to **STRESS**, intentional exercise or just life in general.

Keep in mind our objective is to focus the 16 hours you have each day to:

- Optimize simple components of your life to reduce Inflammation and Oxidation.
- Improve the markers of your health such as: CRP, HDL, Triglyceride, Insulin Resistance, Recovery Rates, and Body Composition.

What is your current program of Physical Activity and Exercise doing for you?

The Metafit 360 Solution to Overtraining

Feel Good Exercise monitored by personal and group tracking technologies and regular HRV readings, not to mention beginning C-Reactive Protein Blood Test. Proper exercise bouts should be *stimulating* – NOT- *Overly Destructive*. Remember Goldilocks and the Three Bears:

- *"This porridge is too hot!"* she exclaimed. So, she tasted the porridge from the second bowl.
- *"This porridge is too cold,"* she said. So, she tasted the last bowl of porridge.
- *"Ahhh, this porridge is just right,"* she said happily and she ate it all up.

M360 is the *Ahhhhh* in your lifestyle of- exercise, diet and stress management.

Our #1 Objective is to Improve your Fat Metabolism

The rate of fat oxidation during your exercise is determined by:

1. **The availability of fatty acids**
2. **The rate of carbohydrate utilization**

Both absolute and relative (i.e. % of mhr/reference point) exercise intensities play important roles in the regulation of our substrate metabolism (fuel selection).

While exercise intensity determines the percentage of carbohydrate and fat oxidized by working muscles, absolute work (load) rate determines the total quantity of fuel required.

- As relative exercise intensity is increased, there is a:
  - **Decrease in the percentage of total energy that is derived from fat oxidation.**
  - **Increase in energy provided by carbohydrate oxidation.**
- During *moderately strenuous exercise* of an intensity that can be maintained for 90 minutes or longer (approximately 50-80% of MHR), there is a **progressive decline** in the proportion of energy derived from muscle glycogen and a **progressive increase** in plasma fatty acid oxidation.

Do you Monitor the Markers of Intensity, Duration and Frequency?

If you do not monitor these markers, then **HOW** do you know your workout is effective?

What are you doing and why?

As we become metabolically **FAT ADAPTED** via- adaptations that are induced with the proper intensity, duration and frequency of endurance exercise training results in a developed metabolic capacity or ability to spare (minimize use) carbohydrate during exercise, with an increased proportion of the energy being provided by much more efficient **fat oxidation**.

Fat Oxidation and Fat Adaption is a Key Re-Occurring Theme of M360

Research proves, without doubt that trained individuals oxidize more fat and less carbohydrate, than untrained subjects when performing sub-maximal work of the same- absolute intensity.

The purpose of ATP and FFA training, in and Un-Fed State, in the **FEEL GOOD** intensity zone- is to **OPTIMIZE** your **Fat Burning Capacity**. This will not only increase aerobic performance capacity, it will also set the metabolic stage for less Inflammation and Oxidation to occur at the cellular level.

This increased capacity to utilize energy from fat conserves crucial muscle and liver glycogen stores and can contribute to increased endurance and less Free Radical- Oxidative Stress.

Fat Burning Benefits

Further benefits of the enhanced lipid metabolism accompanying -**Feel Good**- aerobic exercise training is **decreased cardiac risk factors**.

M360 Targeted Exercise training results in optimal levels of:

- **hs - C Reactive Protein (CRP)**
- **Less triglycerides**
- **Lower insulin resistance**
- **Increased high density lipoprotein (HDL) cholesterol.**

So **HOW** Do we produce the Perfect Exercise Lifestyle Program?

Common sense and science will guide us if you seek the truth. There can be no lies, deceptions or half truths. Just like it is important to define the components of your lifestyle, it is critical to define the components of your health and performance that you want your efforts to improve and support over time. You must take it upon yourself to identify these components we are helping you to recognize and adopt. You must then put your action up against biomarkers and behaviors you will hold yourself accountable to for the **REST OF YOUR LIFE!**

What are the components of Physical Activity and Exercise that drive you? _____

What did you come up with? _____

The sad truth is most people have NO IDEA why they are working out, or what their effort will affect. It is **CRITICAL** to define goals and markers **BEFORE** any activity or program is started.

There is **POWER** in **WHY**, and **POWER** in **WHAT** we define and **CHOOSE** to do!

Leash yourself to that **POWER** and **SUCCEED!** Lollygag and wander through the fitness gadgets- gizmo's and garbage programs out there and you will fail. It is a matter of statistical fact.

Worthy Components we will help you Target & Improve

How about Breathing? What kind of Exercise program starts without breathing? Kind of hard to do anything without Oxygen isn't it?

Breathing is critical to life

Breathing is critical to your ability to produce energy. Breathing is the one thing you can affect **RIGHT NOW**, in your next breath. I want you to take over a mindset of relaxation and release. Any "Competent" exercise program will start with a course on breathing and make it known that the underlying purpose of activity is to help you **Breathe Easier**!

Relaxation is <u>NOT</u> something that you do.

- Relaxation is a natural response that you **<u>ALLOW</u>** to happen.
- Relaxation is what is left when you stop creating tension.
- Remember a few pages back the 3 contractions of movement and muscle stress?
- Relaxation and Exercise starts with releasing that tension.
- Let go of your contraction
  - Let your eyes go soft
  - Relax your face
  - Just let go of your mind-body tensions.

Relaxation is allowing your internal pace to slow down, allow the waves of breath to ebb and flow. Focus your attention on the flow of your breath, in and out - while you allow each breath to carry away your tension. Allow the waves of breath to wash away the tension. Even take a moment to purposely **TENSE** your diaphragm to feel the **TENSION**, squeeze and feel your internal abdominal pressure - only so you can **FEEL** the **RELEASE**- when you relax, and let go.

Efficient Breathing is a matter of <u>MORE</u> for <u>LESS</u>

As you relax, let your lungs **FILL** with a deep **BELLY BREATH**. Learn to feel the relaxation of these deep belly breaths that come from a fully relaxed diaphragm.

- **M360** is all about oxygenating the cells of your body to- optimize the creation of energy, boundless relaxed and sustainable energy.

- If you will truly learn to relax, release, and focus- as we pinpoint a lifestyle you can sustain. You will find exercise and physical activity Nirvana!

Proper breathing is your best friend as you perform meaningful exercise routines and joyful physical activities. As you find the harmony within the framework of your mind, your body and the components of your lifestyle you will achieve your optimal metabolic health and self respect. It all starts with your **NEXT** breath! Everything **M360** proposes keeps in mind metabolic health, and learning to:

Release and Perform vs. Grind and Destroy

Think about it a little deeper... nothing happens without oxygen, your ability to relax, optimize and understand the flow of air in and out of your body is critical and fundamental to everything you do!

Please take a moment to go to our podcast on Google Play or iTunes, under Power 2 Learn and listen to our podcast: **Power 2 Learn**

"12 minutes to unleash the Power of your Next Breath".

Summary of Breathing Dynamics and CPET

Breathing is a universal wave flow of air going in and gas coming out of your lungs. I have been through and recommend CPET or Cardio Pulmonary Exercise Testing to demonstrate the function of breathing. We call the test Gas Exchange as CPET is really just the measure of Oxygen (O2) being extracted from air being- inhaled- and Gas (CO2) being −exhaled-. This gas exchange tells us how efficient you are at supplying oxygen to the cells of your body as you remove gas. This exchange is what keeps you alive and provides cellular respiration for life.

Life is a <u>FLOW</u> of Mind and Breath in time with Action and Circumstance

This universal wave flow is easy to picture in your mind. Picture a balloon that you blow up to its maximum. Your vital capacity (VC) is the maximum capacity of your lungs when they are fully inflated. Like the balloon there is a certain amount of pressure that assists the flow of Oxygen into the body and Gas out of the body.

For sake of example let's say your maximum inhalation capacity or Vital Capacity (VC) is 5 liters of air:

- If you exhale 1 liter -you can inhale 1 liter - if you exhale 3 liters, you can inhale up to 3 liters.
- My point here is to show you the importance of exhaling.

Exhaling is the most controllable portion of the universal wave flow of breathing. M360 will help you learn to utilize your ability to exhale- to relax, release, and better ventilate your metabolic need for oxygen- and the removal of CO_2 gas.

How important is your breathing rate, depth and rhythm?

Heart rate increases slightly when we breathe in (inhalation), and decreases when we breathe out (exhalation) in a phenomenon known as respiratory sinus arrythmia (RSA).

Heart and Breathing Rates

Our pulse- or heart rate (HR) is the number of times our heart beats in a minute. Resting heart rate varies with age and level of physical fitness, with normal resting pulse ranging from:

- **60 to 80 beats per minute in most moderately healthy people**

Your breathing rate is measured in a similar manner, with an average resting rate of:

- **12 to 20 breaths per minute**

Our heart beats roughly 4 times for every breath we take, so as intensity of activity goes up so does our rate of breathing along with increased heart rate. The healthier and fitter you get the more in tune you will become with both thresholds of respiration and heart rate.

Breathing and Physical Activity

Physical activity increases your body's energy requirements. The most efficient way to meet these needs involves the use of oxygen to break down fat and glucose. The more oxygen you can uptake and utilize to produce energy the fitter you are. I once asked **Dr. Vigil his definition of "Fitness"**:

"Tim, since we are aerobes- living on a oxygen planet- our metabolisms are Oxygen Dependent, so the answer to -what is fitness- has to be the individual's ability to uptake and utilize Oxygen to create human energy to fund movement"

Based on this Definition of Fitness: How <u>FIT</u> are <u>YOU</u>?

The objective for our program and our focus on the first 3 metabolic thresholds is to improve your ability to improve and optimize your energy/workload at each of these metabolic thresholds, while reducing overall stress- including Oxidative Stress and your Inflammatory Response. This alone is a true life changer away from the causes of Chronic Disease and your own wonderful healthspan and decreased morbidity.

Here is an example what 5-weeks of **M360** can do for an average individual.

Simple FFA (70%) and ATP Threshold (80%) test before and after 5-week, 15-Modality program:

Test 20 minute FTP @ 70%   **Before: 90 watts**   **After: 110 watts**
Test 20 minute FTP @ 80%   **Before: 110 watts**   **After: 140 watts**

What this means in simple terms is a reduction of stress at same workload or output. **More for less!** Keep in mind this is not just a test for cyclist who live and breathe performance in terms of **POWER**, it is also a test of **VITALITY** and **FUNCTION** for **ALL PEOPLE**. Think of yourself or someone you have known that had great power and athleticism while young and competing, then as they aged and got away from the regiments of training and a disciplined lifestyle, you witness their **POWER** and **MUCHO GUSTO** slip to moderate **VITALITY** then sadly to loss of **FUNCTION** and on to a **NURSING HOME** and Delayed Suffering in a state of elongated **MORBIDITY**.

Do <u>NOT</u> let your FLAME flicker and cease to burn

This is our **M360 PASSION**; it starts and ends with the health and performance of:

- Our **Cells**
- Our **Metabolism**
- Our **Mitochondria**!!

Embrace the truth, drop the **FAD** and let's learn together, let us explore the wonder of **HEALTH** and **Metabolic Fitness for Life.**

All points of each section of this book and program point in the same direction.

- Lifestyle to allow for Physical Activity and Exercise,
- Diet that Supports Exercise and Physical Activities (What you DO!)

- Stress management that allows you to **SUSTAIN** and **REPEAT** success.

Cellular Power, Vitality and Function are based in efficacy of movement

People who once spent 70% of their max heart rate and ventilation rates to get 90 watts of power output, after just 5-weeks are getting 110-120 watts, the equivalent of getting for example $120.00 per unit of work instead of $90.00 per unit. This is huge as it also lowers overall Stress in the testable form of:

- **CRP, which is directly linked to lowering:**
- **Cardio Vascular Disease (CVD) as well as:**
- **Down regulating the pace of aging.**

The result of increasing your cardiorespiratory output is like tossing a stone into a calm pond. The ripples that cascade throughout your life are priceless.

Cardiorespiratory Fitness (CRF) -Clinical Marker of Health and Performance

Research has firmly established that low levels of cardiorespiratory fitness (CRF) are associated with a high risk of cardiovascular disease, all-cause mortality, and mortality rates attributable to various cancers.

Cardio Respiratory Fitness is a Predictor of Health Outcomes

- CRF reflects the integrated ability to transport oxygen from the atmosphere to the mitochondria to create the energy needed to perform physical work.
- Cardio Respiratory Fitness quantifies the **Functional Capacity** of an individual and is dependent on a linked chain of processes that include:

- ○ **Functional Capacity** to ventilate and diffuse Oxygen
- ○ **Functional Capacity** of the right and left ventricular function of your heart. (both systole and diastole),
- ○ **Functional Capacity** of your Ventricular-arterial coupling, the ability of the vasculature to accommodate and efficiently transport blood from the heart to supply oxygen requirements that keep you alive and thriving.
- ○ **Functional Capacity** of your muscle cells and mitochondria to receive and use the oxygen and nutrients delivered by the blood to efficiently produce **ENERGY** for you to live and perform better.

Clearly, your Cardio Respiratory Function (CRF) is directly related to the integrated function of numerous systems, and it is considered a reflection of total body health.

How is your Cardiorespiratory Fitness?

Metafit Cardio Respiratory Fitness Testing & Reference Point Training (RPT)

M360 Submaximal Exercise Testing is performed on clinical grade -smart trainers with correlations of CRF being derived directly from the relation between the incremental responses of **HEART RATE** in relation to **WORK RATE** (Power Output) HR/WR.

In this case sustainable average **4-min - 20-min Power Outputs** (Wattage) are measured in terms of average:

- **Beats per minute (bpm)**
- **Percentage % of Maximum Heart Rate**
- **Percentage % of Max Vo2**

Typically, **2 sub-maximal work rates are performed**, with measures of steady-state HR being recorded after 4 minutes and 20 minutes, at a personalized sub-maximal work rate in the **70%** to **80%** mhr work range.

1. 70% representing the upper limits of your FFA capacity
2. 80% representing the upper limits of your ATP capacity

(Aerobic Transition Point)

Example: I will use my own numbers to show you how we categorize specific 20' sub max test that will determine my first 2-Aerobic Training Zones. With me being the patient/athlete at age 60 and a tested maximum HR of 166 bpm the results are logged and categorized in **3 Target Training Zones as follows**:

Zone #1- Intensity and Effect

FFA- short for **Free Fatty Acid** utilization:

- **Low intensity/longer duration aerobic activities** that target and promote metabolic **Fat Adaption**.
- **Heart rate monitors are used to measure intensity kept between 50%-70%** mhr. I do these with my wife at 50% to keep her at 70%, so it is a long fun day of riding together and we both target Fat Adaption and better allocation of metabolic energy. We ride 40-100 mile single day rides once a week at these intensity rates. Keep in mind the fitter you are you can take FFA up to **75%**, so I use **70%** as a medium reference. You may peak FFA @ **65%**?
- **These sessions are usually done in a Fasted – Un-Fed State** for up to 8 hours- as in a 100 mile- low intensity bike ride. Done in and out of facility.
- **FFA should represent 45%-65% of your total weekly time spent in activity or exercise.** Example would be 4.5 to 6.5 hours of every 10 hours you spend in activity to promote health and metabolism.

- **This metabolic zone is the <u>Energy Base</u> to Everything You DO!**

Sample Range of Intensity using my own numbers for a 60 year old athlete:

- **20' @ 230 watt avg.** currently cost me and average of 116 bpm or 70% of my mhr of 167 bpm. Performed on our Stages Indoor Bikes w/Power Meter.

Note: Stages is the official sponsor of power meters for Team Sky!

- **For 20 minutes** in my current state of fitness I can ride an average of **230 watts** at an average **metabolic cost of 70%** mhr or 116 bpm.
- **The goal of my training** is to increase the wattage at 70% incrementally to reflect 240w-245w avg. etc.
- **As I age into my 70's and 80's** the goal will be to maintain and sustain, Power, Vitality and Function (PVF). These numbers become my yardstick of aging and performance. We will see a slip in individuals from **Power** to **Vitality** on to **Function** and then ultimately we all lose function and die.
- Our goal is to **GET STRONGER NOW**! Our goal is to slow down the inevitable - often un-talked about- rate of your slide to morbidity and death.
- **PVF is your Life Force** and you would be well advised to keep close tabs on it:
  - **Know it**
  - **Honor it**
  - **Love it**
  - **Improve it!**

Zone #2- Intensity and Effect

ATP- Short for **Aerobic Transition Point**:

- Medium Intensity/Moderate Duration 70%-80% mhr
- Often referred to as Tempo work, done in and Aerobic State
- Objective of ATP training is to improve Aerobic Capacity.
- Focus will be improving Neuro Muscular Facilitation (NMF) @ ATP. Simply put the objective is to improve your Efficiency of Movement, which in turn will reduce your Metabolic Cost of that movement.
- ATP will be done in 4 minute – 20 minute durations with the focus on Power output at or below 80% of your maximum heart rate. Again you may be fitter and 85% may be more accurate for the limits of ATP or less fit and it may be 75%. I use 80% as a medium level transition point.
- ATP should represent 25%-30% of total activity time spent focused on quality movement in a relaxed state specific to what you are doing- paddling, riding, running, swimming, etc.
- **ATP to shed Fat Mass** should be done in a Metabolically **Un-Fed** state, preferably in the morning after an intermittent fast of 12-14 hours.
- **ATP in a Fed State** would be done to focus on improving **Power Output** during a more competitive time of year or when you feel the need for a little feeding to stimulate a special testing of your aerobic capacity.

Sample Range of Intensity @ ATP maximum of 80% using my own numbers for a 60 year old athlete: Again, test was done on Stages Indoor Bike with Stages Power Meters and Garmin (ANT) Heart Rate Monitor.

- **20' @ 252 watt avg.** currently cost me and average of 132 bpm or 80% of my mhr of 167 bpm.

- **For 20 minutes in my current state of fitness** I can ride an average of **252 watts** at an average **metabolic cost of 80%** mhr or 132 bpm.
- **The goal of my training is** to increase the wattage at 80% incrementally to reflect **260w-265w** avg. etc.
- **As I age into my 70's and 80's** the goal will be to maintain and sustain, Power, Vitality and Function (PVF).
- **PVF is your Life Force** and you would be well advised to keep close tabs on it, know it, honor it, love it, and improve it!
- **What will my 20 minute average power output be at age 80?**

What will your 20 minute power output be in terms of wattage, at 80 yrs old?

Zone #3- Intensity and Effect

LBP- Short for <u>Lactate Balance Point</u>:

- Intensity "run-ups" or "tempo@" 1'- 20' duration 80%-90% mhr depending on fitness. The fitter you are the higher you can go in terms of heart rate vs. onset of blood lactate accumulation (OBLA)
- Often referred to as Lactate Threshold work, done in and Anaerobic State
- LBP training objective is to improve **Aerobic Power** and **Aerobic Ceiling**
- Focus will be improving **POWER @ LBP.** Simply put the objective is to improve your Power of point of Lactate Balance just **"BEFORE"** getting into deep **Metabolic Acidosis.**
- LBP will be done in 1 minute – 20 minute durations with the focus on Power output at or below 90% of your maximum heart rate. Just below OBLA!
- **OBLA is:** Onset of Blood Lactate Accumulation. Think of Lactate like water pouring into a bath tub with the drain open.

Just enough water (Lactate) coming into the tub (Working Muscle) as going out the drain (Being Utilized). The tub never runs over, in perfect energy balance.

- LBP should represent 0%-5% of total activity time spent focused on quality movement in a relaxed but **POWERFUL** state specific to what you are doing- paddling, riding, running, swimming, etc.
- **LBP to shed Fat Mass** should be done in a Metabolically **Un-Fed** state, preferably in the morning after an intermittent fast of 12-14 hours.
- **LBP in a Fed State** would be done to focus on improving **Power Output** during a more competitive time of year or when you feel the need for a little feeding to stimulate a special testing of your Aerobic Ceiling or Balance of POWER @ LBP.

Sample Range of Intensity @ LBP maximum of 90% using my own numbers for a 60 year old athlete:

- **15' @ 272 watt avg.** currently cost me and average of 145 bpm or 87.3% of my mhr of 166 bpm. I did this in a Zwift Race Environment making it interesting and motivational. My watts per Kilo for 15'= 3.4wpk. This becomes my training marker for this 5% of my total **M360** program.
- **For 15 minutes in my current state of fitness** I can ride an average of **272 watts** at an average **metabolic cost of 87.3%** mhr or 145 avg. bpm.
- **The goal of my training is** to increase the wattage at 88% incrementally to reflect **280w-285w** avg. etc.
- **As I age into my 70's and 80's** the goal will be to maintain and sustain, power, vitality and function (PVF). To **SLOW** the inevitable aging process
- **PVF is your Life Force** and you would be well advised to keep close tabs on ALL ASPECTS of it at ALL 3 Levels of our **M360** Program. Know it, honor it, love it, and improve it!

- **What will my 15 minute average <u>LBP</u> power output be at age 80?**

What will your 20 minute power output be in terms of wattage, at 80 yrs old? _____

M360 resistance training is set at **50%/70% RPT** either as free standing sessions or mixed into a circuit. **12-24 reps at 50% 1 rep max** and **6-12 reps at 70% 1 rep max.**

What is your 1 rep max of each of your 6 body parts? _____

Cost of Physical Activity Exercise and Life as a Metabolic Equivalent MET

The **Metabolic Equivalent of Task (MET)**, or simply **metabolic equivalent** is:

- The physiological measure of energy cost for a given physical activity or exercise
- MET is defined as the ratio of metabolic rate referenced to a conventional average rate of 3.5 ml ml/kg/min *milligram per kilogram per minute.

A single MET is the amount of oxygen a person consumes (or the energy expended) per unit (Kg) of body weight during 1-minute of rest. This is your baseline.

- Baseline MET is equal to about 3.5 milliliters (ml) of oxygen consumption per kilogram (kg) of body weight per minute or 1 kilocalorie (kcal) per kg of body weight per hour.

When using METs as an intensity guide **make sure you understand** at what intensity you need to be exercising. As a general rule:

- 4–6 METs is considered moderate intensity;
- Greater than 10 METs is considered vigorous activity.

With all this said, it is just base information for you to be aware of when you hear the term METs as a measure of Physical Activity.

We will be using the relationship of our tested Energy Transition Thresholds of **FFA, ATP** and **LPB** (Higher Intensity Interval Training) to determine the correlation between workload and metabolic cost as an expression of %Percentage of MHR and % Percentage of Functional Threshold Power for 1'-2'-4'-10'-20' and 1-hour of Functional Power.

- All Sessions will be automatically posted to our global metabolic app upon completion of session to reflect your entire lifestyle from:
  - **Sleep**
  - **Stress**
  - **Power**
  - **Speed**
  - **Pace**
  - **Calories**
  - **Heart Rate from Resting to:**
    - **FFA**
    - **ATP**
    - **LBP.**

To simplify this portion of **M360** it will be fun to improve your workload at same metabolic output.

- Remember our goal is not to **PUSH** you harder and **PAIN** you,
- Our goal is to get **more out of you** at **Same Cost**.
- We literally will **LOWER** your **COST** of **LIVING** in terms of **Metabolic Cost**- wear and tear we will summarize as **STRESS!**

M360 will increase your Aerobic **Power/Vitality/Function** and **Lower Stress!**

STOP RIGHT NOW! Think a minute about what it would truly mean to your performance and life to improve all 10 markers of your health.

These changes to our select biomarkers will cascade and ripple across the metaphoric pond of your life and contribute to the reduction of Inflammation an Oxidation, and by doing so reduce, even eliminate and reverse the conditions of Chronic Disease.

Constructing activities outside and in our exercise facility that develop your aerobic power and reduce stress is one of my specialties as I love constructing these routines for myself. There is an endless variety of routines we will engage in that will **STIMULATE** metabolic health, monitor recovery and increase your metabolic fitness for life.

Autonomic Nervous System is the King of your Cardio Workout

Our autonomic nervous system (ANS) is divided into 2 distinct modes; both have a direct role in our physical response to stress:

- **Sympathetic nervous system** (SNS)
- **Parasympathetic nervous system** (PNS)

When the body is stressed, the SNS generates what is known as the **"fight or flight"** response. Energy resources (metabolic functions) are shifted into high gear upon the perception of threat and danger. Our Fight or Flight mechanisms goes into a state of high alert until the perceived danger passes. At this point the Sympathetic Nervous system *should deactivate* and the parasympathetic nervous system *should activate*, but does it? This on and off adaptation is something we should be more aware of and better able to control. For this reason our M360 sessions conduct ANS training sessions.

The SNS signals the adrenal glands to release hormones called:

- **Adrenalin**
- **Cortisol**

These hormones cause:

- The heart to beat faster
- Respiration rate to increase
- Blood vessels in the arms and legs to dilate
- Digestive process to change
- Glucose levels (sugar energy) in the bloodstream to increase to deal with the emergency.

In order to prepare our bodies to respond to an emergency situation of short term- acute stressors- the response of our **Sympathetic Nervous System (SNS)** very rapid. Once the crisis is over, our nervous system should return to a Parasympathetic, unstressed state.

Chronic stress (experiencing stressors over a prolonged period of time); will result in a long-term drain on our body. Constant **"Over Awareness"** and **"Over Response"** of our **SNS** continues to trigger metabolic reactions, and with it excessive/needless wear-and-tear on our body.

It's not so much **WHAT** chronic stress does to the nervous system, but **HOW** continuous over-activation of the nervous system affects other bodily systems that become problematic. This excessive and often needless stressing of our metabolic reaction becomes yet another source of ROS and Oxidative Stress.

Our goal is simple: make everyone who seeks us out, aware of needless stress and arm them with ways to reduce it.

- What are your Trigger Points?
- What can you eliminate from your life as a source of undue stress?

We Need to Recover Between Workouts to Avoid Chronic Inflammation

There is no doubt that the proper feel good exercise can reduce inflammation but the wrong excessive intensity exercise can also increase inflammation. The difference is, when proper intensity physical activity and exercise is done regularly over the long term, it will decrease chronic –or– systemic silent inflammation. Mild oxidative stress from moderate reference point training (RPT) forces our body to build up antioxidant defenses. This is indicated in studies showing proper exercise programs that take metabolic science into action:

- **Reduce inflammatory markers such as C-reactive protein**

Acute inflammation can become chronic, so part of the equation involves exercising in such a way as to:

- Avoid turning those acute bouts of inflammation into a chronic one. I spent 12 years at Therafit stressing the importance of recovery — *especially* when doing HIIT — and this is precisely why.
- If you over-train, you typically will end up doing more harm than good, as your body needs to recuperate from the damage (inflammation) incurred during your workout. It is referred to as the Super Compensation Model.
- See some of the Blogs on various topics at our website: **www. metafit.life**

M360 Feel Good Exercise for a REASON by personal Reference Point:

Effective exercise is the introduction of workload that initiates a temporary, but powerful inflammatory response.

M360 sessions are a combination of:

- **STIMULATING** Load and Recover activities done in 3 primary zones:
  - **FFA** activities are a variety of **FUN** activities done in and **Un-Fed** State below 65% of MHR in durations of 2-hours or more against a backdrop of a Functional Diet to support target objectives.
  - **ATP** Aerobic Transition Point Training @ 65%-75% of MHR Higher
  - **LBP** sessions are done in small pieces of intermittent nature building up to what we call Lactate Dynamics of coming up to Onset of Blood Lactate Accumulation and then backing off to lower intensity only to come back up again and again like a stair case. "Higher" Intensity Interval Training (**HIIT**) @ or "Up to" 90% of MHR.
  - **50/70** sessions of resistance training always allow plenty of rest with focus on as perfect **Neuro Muscular Facilitation as possible. Perfect Biomechanics.**

All Modalities allow for plenty of recovery time against a backdrop of lots of FFA

Intensities, Durations & Frequencies that benefit Fat Oxidation

It is well-established that whole body **FAT OXIDATION** increases with exercise intensity up 50-70% of MHR, but decreases at higher exercise intensity above 75%-80% of MHR. Fat oxidation (Lypolysis) shifts to sugar utilization (Glycolysis) as intensity increases

The exercise intensity at which maximal fat oxidation rates occur varies according to training status, sex, and mode of exercise.

M360 Focus is on Sub maximal "<u>FEEL GOOD</u>" Exercise

It is well-established that endurance training increases fat oxidation during sub maximal exercise. These adaptations have commonly been observed in response to low to moderate intensity (50-70% of MHR) exercise training programs lasting 5-10 weeks.

Studies show that daily low to moderate intensity training sessions (2 hr/day) induce an increase in fat oxidation during exercise within 7-10 days.

The effect of 50/70 resistance training of fat oxidation has not been as well-studied as the effects of endurance training. Most studies in this area have measured the acute effects of resistance exercise on fat oxidation in the period **after** exercise. Key here is whether you **FEED** the **SESSION (anabolism)** or allow the Fat Utilization to provide the post exercise energy via Fat Stores **(catabolism).** Fat oxidation is enhanced in the **UN- FED** post-exercise period. We will teach how to cycle these metabolic states to optimize metabolic fitness for life.

What are the 24 hour effects of M360 Exercise on Fat Oxidation

Macronutrient intake will also affect fat oxidation. Carbohydrate overfeeding- creates an immediate and distinctive shift in fuel utilization:

- Suppressing the oxidation of fat
- Increasing carbohydrate oxidation, and energy expenditure.

Diet and Exercise affect FAT OXIDATION

Increasing the intake of dietary fat from 40% to 70% causes a substantial reduction in carbohydrate utilization while increasing fat oxidation. **Note:** we will cover this in detail in section 3 on Diet and Nutrition.

Heart Rate Variability (HRV) & Autonomic Nervous System (ANS) health

American Heart Association data suggest that low heart rate variability (HRV) (high stress) is associated with a higher risk of death in patients with heart disease and in elderly subjects and with a higher incidence of **Coronary Heart Disease (CHD)** in the general population.

Subjects with low HRV had a high cardiovascular risk profile and an elevated risk of incident CHD and death. The increased risk of death could not be attributed to a specific cause and could not be explained by other risk factors.

- Low HRV is associated with increased risk of CHD and death from several causes. It is hypothesized that low HRV is a marker of less favorable health.
- Heart rate variability (HRV) decreases under situations of stress, either emotional or physical, whereas it increases with rest.
- HRV is considered a noninvasive marker of autonomic nervous system function.

Heart Rate Variability- Stress and Mortality Rates

A population study of middle-aged men and women with low HRV, as determined from a 2 minute test, had an adverse cardiovascular risk profile and elevated risk of death from all causes, including cancer, and of incident CHD. The elevated risk could not be attributed to other risk factors.

- HRV is an important predictor of CHD events.
- Low HRV was a strong predictor of death, but at this writing- because of the limited number of cases, the relation with specific causes of death could not be analyzed.
- In a prospective study of middle-aged there was a strong association between low HRV and death from all causes, including cancer. The results of other studies are in line with these findings.

- It may be hypothesized that low HRV is an indicator of poor general health.

What is the average- of your RHR over the last 30 days? _____

Risks of all-cause, and specifically- cardiovascular mortality, are much higher in people with elevated resting heart rate (RHR). One of the biggest predictors of all-cause and cardiovascular mortality - is our resting heart rate! Every 10 beat increment of RHR above 60 bpm is a biomarker indicative of an imbalance between the vagal and the sympathetic tone, or a dysfunctional autonomic nervous system. The higher our resting heart rate in 10 beat increments above 60 bpm (70-80-90) there is a direct detrimental proclivity toward a progression of coronary atherosclerosis.

Resting Heart Rate RHR can be a sign of sympathetic hyperactivity and a poor parasympathetic tonus. Dysfunctional autonomic balance can disrupt many metabolic functions and lead to a decline in performance. PLEASE be aware of this, and make an effort to discover what components of your life are affecting activation of parasympathetic and deactivation of sympathetic. I have noticed night time eating close to bedtime will elevate my resting heart rate.

Tracking Trending Heart Rate

I use my Garmin Fenix 5x to track my 24/7 HR trend with automatically downloads to my Garmin Connect App. This gives me a clear 30,000 ft perspective of RHR and my life stress. I am currently trending around 45-50 bpm RHR. In the process of writing this book I myself have become more aware of stress and how to reduce it with many tools you will find in Section 4. I have seen it trend down from the mid 50's to low 50's/high 40's. Awareness works!

Resting Heart Rate and who should be considered at risk?

Under resting conditions, the adult human heart beats at about 70 to 75 bpm, and the heart rate tends to decrease with age. Women generally have a 3-7 bpm higher heart rate than men.

The normal limits of resting heart rate are nominally between 60 and 100 bpm. Many studies have found the following RHR specifics:

- RHR above 80-85 bpm may imply a notable increase in cardio vascular (CV) risk.
- On the other had rates lower than 60 bpm have been shown to be protective against cardiovascular disease.

Studies indicate there is a significant-increased risk of CVD, with heart rates higher than 80-85 bpm. If you are 60 -80 you need to be asking yourself what direction am I going, UP or DOWN.

What is your average resting Heart Rate? _____

Post Exercise Recovery Rate (PERR) Tracking for Training Sessions:

1- Minute of Recovery and Mortality Rates

- The first minute of post exercise recovery is the most critical!
- Post activity- your heart rate should experience an abrupt drop in the first minute.
- This Post Exercise Recovery Rate (PERR) not only indicates fitness level it also gives us a window of warning to potential heart problems, and is considered a prime marker of mortality rate in humans.

In an October 1999 article in "The New England Journal of Medicine," a study performed by the Cleveland Clinic Foundation classified a heart rate decrease of **12 beats or less** in the first minute as abnormal.

The study also reported that people with an **abnormal decline in heart rate had a greater chance of mortality** in the subsequent six years due to heart problems.

What is your 1-Minute, Post Max Heart Rate Recovery rate? _____

2- Minute Post Exercise Recovery Rate

Our heart rate 2- minutes after exercise is referred to as our recovery heart rate. 2- Minute PERR is the most common measurement to determining cardiovascular fitness. To test for improvements:

- Record maximum heart rate in BPM during exercise test, then record recovery heart rate at the two-minute post exercise mark. i.e.150max 100 @ 2' = 50 beat 2' PERR recovery rate

12 years of 1 minute PERR Therafit Records in BPM Post <u>Max</u> Exercise:

A+ >45

A 40+

B 30+

C 20+

D 15+

F <12 go see Cardiologist Immediately!!

What is your 1 and 2 Minute Post Exercise -Recovery Rate? _____

- The fitter you are, the faster you **recover**, it is that simple!
- Within the **first minute after we stop exercising (post exercise)**; our heart rate should come down a minimum of 20

beats minute, with a drop of less than 12 beats a minute- being considered **very abnormal**. This is critical to your healthspan and longevity. This is a test you can do right now!

- Your **2-minute "recovery heart rate"** is measured as part of our **M360** exercise stress test on a weekly basis during fun feel good physical activities and exercise routines. The 2 minute recovery can be done from a Sub-Max effort, making it more user friendly as a frequent measure of your cardio fitness.
- **Application to athletic performance.**
  - **Question:** Two - 4 minute milers get together and run a simple 5-minute mile together. They both basically jog a 5- minute mile. **Who is fitter?**

Answer: The one who recovers faster and can do it again!

Recovery and **Balance** are two **VERY IMPORTANT** words at **M360**.

Recovery and Balance are both **KEY** to your **Optimum Health** and performance whether you are 87 years old, just trying to function and keep your independence from the dread of a **NURSING HOME**, or whether you are a 19 year old 4:02 Miler trying to break a 4 minute mile and run 3:55 to make the Olympic Team. The basic fundamentals of metabolic health and performance are missing from our Healthcare and Fitness Landscape. **M360** is different; we do everything based on **SCIENCE** and the measurable, documentable biomarkers of your unique and specific genome.

Autonomic Nervous System (ANS) drives Your Metabolism and Performance:

- **UP is (Sympathetic) and DOWN is (Parasympathetic)**

Involuntary body functions are controlled by the autonomic nervous system. The autonomic nervous system has two parts:

- The **<u>sympathetic nervous system</u>** dominates when the body is excited or in a heightened state of alert or fight or flight mode.
- The **<u>parasympathetic nervous system</u>** helps our body to recovery, and returns us to resting our metabolic state of **<u>RECOVERY</u>**. Often referred to as a state of "Rest and Digest".

During exercise our sympathetic nervous system dominates the regulation of body functions. After exercise, the sympathetic nervous system should withdraw and deactivate whilst the parasympathetic nervous system activates and assist our body to return to a resting state of recovery. **M360** will focus on these functions with adapt recover moderate exercise interval sessions.

How well does your body return to a resting state, not only after exercise, but on a daily basis? _____

- Research shows us that post-exercise decrease in our heart rate is almost exclusively controlled by:
  - ○ **parasympathetic reactivation as opposed to:**
  - ○ **sympathetic withdrawal**
- Post-exercise decrease in the heart rate a KEY BIOMARKER of physical fitness and overall cardiovascular health.
- The first minute drop in heart rate is critical. A drop in the heart rate less than **12 bpm** in the first minute of recovery is distinctive warning of cardiovascular impairment. 1 minute post maximal recovery rates below 12 bpm should be an **ALARM** as they are a consistent marker of mortality rates in humans.
- **If you fall in this category we urge you to see a cardiologist immediately for test to reveal potential arterial blockage.**

What is your 1- Minute Post Exercise Recovery Rate again?? _____

If you are truly interested in your long term health and performance you should know this information better than you know your name! It drives me mad that our society focuses on how much we weigh which really tells us nothing!

On the other hand our **1 and 2 minute PERR** tell us everything about our current state of wellness. In-fact, this number is considered one of the most important biomarkers of human mortality rate. In 12 years of teaching at my Therafit studio everyone that had a recovery of less than 12 beats ended up (in hindsight) have a cardiac issue, fortunately most ended in the insertion of a stent and they are still living.

- **Take this Marker VERY SERIOUSLY!!!**

How do you measure recovery from day to day LIFE?

Our answer to the 24 hour clock of recovery from LIFE, just like Post Exercise Recovery from Exercise; is Heart Rate Variability (HRV). Heart rate variability is defined as the standard deviation of the subjects R-R intervals of your heart beat.

- **High variability is indicative of cardiovascular health**
- **Low variability is indicative of cardiovascular impairment**

*Don't be confused by devices like **Garmin** who do a **STRESS TEST**

- **LOW** scores meaning **LOW STRESS,** but **HIGH HRV** and:
- **High** scores meaning **HIGH STRESS,** meaning **LOW HRV**

Using a state of the art **Garmin Fenix 5x** my average morning HRV score is, on average, less than or equal to **20** on a scale of 1-100 (1 being High HRV and 100 being Low HRV). I track this daily and keep in mind the whole objective of this metric is to manage your stress levels.

Keep in mind what is killing us from section #1. The answer is chronic conditions brought on by chronic inflammation and oxidation. Show me chronic inflammation and oxidation and I will show you chronic disease. In this I will give highlight to this fact:

Show me Chronic Inflammation and Oxidation in an Olympic Athlete and I will show you poor performance, injury and illness!

Nobody can escape the basic human need of our metabolism, our need for efficient energy and optimum mitochondrial function. Mess that up and the whole house of cards will cave in on you. Remember our objective? Answer: Mitochondrial Fitness for Life (Metafit.life or **M360**. We are NOT a SPIN class. WE are NOT a GYM. WE are a Systematic Group of Like minded Champions of Health looking to acquire and maintain:

Metabolic Fitness for LIFE!

Be it Lifestyle, Diet or Stress Management – We all have OPTIONS of Exercise

Parasympathetic reactivation is slower after high intensity interval than after moderate continuous and exercise.

Too many programs are far too intense and as a result, they are destructive to metabolic health and long-term performance- **NOT** what we want to experience for long-term health.

- Our focus at **M360** is on the **parasympathetic** portion of the autonomic nervous system and not so much on lactate threshold performance. Remember our focus is Metabolic Health & Fitness for LIFE.
- A Key Focus of **M360** is to improve Vagal Tone:
  - **Vagal tone** is the parasympathetic nerve activation used in controlling/lowering our heart rate. Good Vagal tone would mean effective activation of our parasympathetic nervous system.

What is the condition of your post-exercise autonomic shift?

- **HRRec** is more indicative of our **vagal tone** (sympathetic release):
- **HRV** is indicative of our **parasympathetic activation**.

Distinct shifts in our autonomic function are valuable, as they are great markers of our overall training status and cardio respiratory fitness as well as our status of potential overtraining. Overtraining will produce a higher trend in Resting Heart Rate and HRV, when you see this on your tracking device it is time to back off a bit.

We suggest a good Heart Rate Monitor with a community mobile app. We use Garmin with Garmin Connect and Strava to record and log our training diary to learn from. Keep in mind it is not about what you do in a day as much as it is about your **TREND** over **TIME!**

M360 will improve HRV and HRRec while lowering Blood Pressure

- <u>**It is important to understand the Dynamics of Blood Pressure**</u>

Each heartbeat has two basic parts:

1. **Diastole (di-AS-toe-lee)** (relax/recover phase): During diastole our hearts relax and begin to fill with blood!
2. **Systole (SIS-toe-lee)** (contract/pump phase): At the end of diastole, our hearts contract (atrial systole) and pump blood into the ventricles.

I have always associated this process with breathing **IN** and **OUT**. Gas Exchange, relax and dilate followed by contract and exhale or discharge.

It is Important to Track our Pulse and Metabolism 24/7/365

We strongly recommend that each of our program participants have a newer Garmin device such as the Vivo Active HR, Forerunner 235, Fenix 5 or higher. All are a justified investment into the future of your health which makes the relative expense minimal. This device will live and breathe with you on a 24 hour tracking system- your personal metabolic fitness for life buddy. This will give you that 30,000 ft trending overview of lifestyle patterns that are critical toward metabolic success. Body weight for example it is what it is on any given day, what is most important is the question of what direction is it trending- **Up** or **Down?** The same is true with RHR and so many other biomarkers.

Dynamics of our Cardiovascular System

Our heart's electrical system controls all the events that occur when our heart pumps blood. The electrical system also is called the cardiac conduction system. If you've ever seen the heart test called an EKG (electrocardiogram), you've seen a graphical picture of the heart's electrical activity.

Three main parts make up our heart's electrical system:

1. The sinoatrial (SA) node- located in the right atrium of our heart
2. The atrioventricular (AV) node- located on the interatrial septum close to the tricuspid valve
3. The His-Purkinje system- located along the walls of our heart's ventricle

The Partnership of Oxygen and Nutrients

Your heart and blood vessels are the two elements of your cardiovascular system that work together to providing you with nourishment and oxygen for the organs of your body. The activity of these two elements is also coordinated in the body's response to – **YOU GUESSED** it **STRESS!**

1. **Acute stress** -stress that is short-term such as meeting deadlines, being stuck in traffic or suddenly slamming on the brakes to avoid an accident –causes:

a. An increase in heart rate, stronger contractions of the heart muscle, increased secretion of stress hormones -adrenaline, noradrenaline and cortisol.

b. Blood vessels that direct blood to the large muscles and the heart dilate, thereby increasing the amount of blood pumped to these parts of the body and elevating blood pressure. *This is also known as the fight or flight response.*

c. Once the acute stress episode has passed, the body returns to its normal state.

2. **Chronic stress**, or a constant stress experienced over a prolonged period of time, can contribute to long-term problems for heart and blood vessels.

a. The consistent and ongoing increase in heart rate, and the elevated levels of stress hormones and of blood pressure, takes a toll on the body.

b. This long-term ongoing stress can increase the risk for hypertension, heart attack or stroke.

Repeated **acute stress** and persistent **chronic stress** may also contribute to **Inflammation** and **Oxidation** in the circulatory system, particularly in the coronary arteries, and this is one pathway that is thought to tie stress to heart attack. It also appears that how a person responds to stress can affect the oxidation of cholesterol.

Liver and Life/Exercise Stress a matter of Managing Stress

When cortisol and epinephrine are released, the liver produces more glucose, a blood sugar that would give you the energy for **"fight or flight"** in an emergency. For most of you, if you don't use all of that extra energy, the body is able to reabsorb the blood sugar, even if you're stressed again and again. But for some people — especially people vulnerable to Type 2 diabetes — that extra blood sugar can mean diabetes.

Who's vulnerable? People who have abused their metabolic systems and are too dependent on their sugar metabolism while testing high for insulin resistance (above 40 via scale).

Studies show that if you learn how to manage stress, and involve yourself in meaningful Physical Activity, supported by Functional Foods -you can control your blood sugar level, sometimes nearly as much as with medication, in a much healthier and sustainable fashion.

Dynamics of Food Timing and Exercise (a case for TRE)

The effect of carbohydrate intake on our fat oxidation is the key to the amount of **FAT** we will burn during and after training sessions.

Consuming as little as 60 g (240 kcals) of carbohydrate during the hour before exercise can reduce lipolysis or **"Ruin Our Quality Fat Oxidation Sessions".** Simply said, sugar will **BLUNT** our opportunity to improve fat adaptation during training. This is referred to as the insulin-induced suppression of lipolysis or Fat Utilization.

If we consume sugar before sessions of exercise- exercising muscle will increase the oxidation of sugar (glycogen) to compensate for the decrease in fat oxidation. The end result is we burn more sugar and less fat, so we effectively **BONK** sooner!

The foods we eat are powerful modulators of fat adaptation or utilization vs. sugar utilization for our mitochondria to make ATP Energy.

Rule of Thumb: Less carbohydrate and calorie restriction in general- will increase fat oxidation, inducing a state of negative fat balance. Give our body the chance to utilize our adiposity (fat stores) by performing longer, less intensity activities in an Un-Fed State. The better we get metabolically at utilize fat as our primary energy substrate for ATP energy- the better fat adapted we will become and with it the less sugar dependent we will be. Free at last of the sugar ball and chain.

FFA Exercise, Nutrition and Timing (More Time Restricted Eating):

It is very well established that fat oxidation during exercise is reduced by carbohydrate consumption prior to or after the exercise. Here are some points for you to consider:

- Fat oxidation/utilization is significant increased when we exercise in a Fasted/UN-Fed State vs. Fed State.
- **M360** sessions and our own physical activities- performed, below 75% of our maximum heart rate for prolonged periods of time - burn more fat and increase aerobic efficiency.
- **M360** utilizes low-to-moderate training intensity because it has been documented to better maximize fat oxidation and aerobic development.
- We recommend that ALL of our aerobic exercise/training suggestions be conducted in a fasted state. We choose low-moderate intensity with more duration and frequency- as compared to higher-training intensities (HIT) that create over-oxidation and metabolic acidosis, often leading to chronic overtraining syndrome, and a cascade of inflammation and oxidation counterproductive to our motivation to produce an **Excellent Metabolism!**

Energy Metabolism Morning vs. Evening

Morning physical activity and exercise produces **greater levels of fat oxidation/utilization** than afternoon and evening activity.

Why?

Because in the morning we are coming off a fasted period of time (sleep), and our blood sugar/insulin levels should be at a daily low. This is the perfect metabolic state to be in- for optimum fat utilization and aerobic ATP energy production. For this reason we front load our sessions into morning at **M360 Clinical Fitness.**

Post Exercise Effect on Energy Metabolism

Research shows that __FAT__ oxidation in the morning- is highest between 6:00am–12:00pm and peaks at its highest level after morning exercise.

Effects of Intensity and Duration on Fat Utilization

Intensity and duration are important factors of fat oxidation exercise and activities.

- Fat oxidation rates are highest as a percentage of total energy between 50% to moderate 70% of max heart rate intensities. We call this FFA Training short for Free Fatty Acid training.
- Fat oxidation rates decrease when intensity goes over 80%. We call this LBP Training short for Lactate Balance Point training
- Maximal rates of fat oxidation/aerobic development occur at intensities between 70%-80% of maximum heart rate in and metabolic Un- Fed State. We call this ATP Training short for Aerobic Transition Point training.

Endurance training induces increased fat oxidation and increase aerobic capacity.

- Consuming carbohydrate before or after exercise reduces our rate of fat utilization/oxidation compared with fasted conditions. For maximum fat utilization, it is best to fast 6 h beyond conclusion of FFA training.

AEROBIC EXERCISE for Aerobes on the Oxygen Planet Earth
Dr. Vigil

Aerobic gains are best made when we perform physical activity using large muscle groups- that can be maintained for long durations (1.5-4 hrs) at a consistent intensity (65%-75%) of MHR (FFA)

Groups of muscles that drive our aerobic activities- depend on our aerobic energy metabolism to convert the substrates into the energy currency of (ATP) adenosine triphosphate from our available of substrates such as:

- Amino acids (Proteins)
- Carbohydrates
- Ketone Bodies
- Fatty Acids (Adiposity/Body Fat)

Aerobic exercise examples include:

- Cycling
- Paddling
- Hiking
- Jogging/long distance running
- Swimming
- Walking
- 50/70 Resistance Training

Our ability to perform aerobic activities is dependent on the condition of our Aerobic Capacity. Our **Aerobic Capacity** is defined as:

- The ability of our cardiorespiratory system to uptake, and utilize oxygen within muscle.
- The gold standard of measuring our aerobic capacity is peak oxygen consumption or (VO_2). Max VO_2 is tested through a variety of procedures via CPET (Cardio Pulmonary Exercise Testing).

ANAEROBIC EXERCISE (AT)

Anaerobic exercise is higher intensity- shorter duration activity, fueled more by substrates like glycogen (sugar) that already exist within our muscle tissue. Anaerobic exercise is oxygen independent. This level of intensity generally starts at or around 75%-85% of our max heart rate. The more aerobically fit we are the higher it starts or in the case of- un-fit, the lower it starts. Since our storage of glycogen in our muscle tissue is limited, the more power or workload we can produce from fat substrate- without going anaerobic- the more work our power we will be able to produce- over the long haul (Longer Duration).

Example:

- Un- fit person may go anaerobic at 75% of Max Heart Rate and start burning much larger quantities of limited muscle glycogen and less and less fat.
- A highly fit and fat adapted person may go to 85% of Max Heart Rate before they start using larger quantities of limited muscle glycogen and less fat.
- The Fit - Fat Adapted person produces more Power or Workload, utilizes less ROS producing sugar, and increases levels of ATP energy by utilizing the much more efficient energy substrate- of body fat- for ATP Fuel.

HOW FAT ADAPTED are YOU?

Anaerobic activities (done in the absence of oxygen) depend on the creation of ATP-*via* a process called glycolysis (Sugar Metabolism). Because Anaerobic Activity produces an excess of lactate, inflammation, oxidative stress and significantly less production of ATP energy than its Fat Burning aerobic counterpart, it is critical to develop our Fat burning Aerobic Capacity.

Listen up please: it is **CRITICAL** to develop our **Aerobic Capacity** and **Ability to utilize Fat for Fuel** (Fat Adapted) to its absolute maximum capacity- to provide the **"Optimum Metabolic Baseline"** we need to efficient fund the energy requirement of our healthy and thriving lifestyle.

Anaerobic Exercises utilizes fast twitch muscles and includes samples:

- Sprinting
- High-intensity interval training (HIIT),
- Power-lifting

Because anaerobic exercise, causes a sustained increase in metabolic acidosis we will cross into this zone less than **5%** o the time at **M360**. This lack of Fat Adaption and lack of specific measured Aerobic work to develop an Optimal Aerobic Capacity is what is **WRONG** with the current landscape of gyms, x fitters and group programs. This **All** or **NOTHING** approach is a waste of your time, money and **METABOLIC HEALH.**

AeT vs. AT why we promote ATP Training

Muscle glycogen- in long term, is the limiting factor to perform high intensity exercise.

- Activities below the AT/LBP (80%-88%mhr) result in a much slower depletion of muscle glycogen than efforts above AT level and tolerable over a longer period of time. This is the TEMPO training zone!
- Training at or near anaerobic threshold level is what we call ATP training. This Sweet Spot –or- Aerobic Transition Point will improve our:
  - ○ Muscle structure
  - ○ Capilarization
  - ○ Oxidative Capacity
  - ○ Substrate Utilization.

The benefits of ATP Training are only achieved when we have systems in place as we do with Stages Cycling and Garmin to monitor and pinpoint exercise intensity. This system allows us to provide evidence based exercise that will target metabolic efficiency by improving aerobic capacity and the efficient ability to utilize and provide ATP energy from a greater and greater volume of body fat.

1. Energy Goes UP
2. Body Fat Stores go DOWN
3. Aerobic Capacity goes UP
4. Inflammation and Oxidation goes DOWN
5. hs-CRP goes DOWN
6. Triglycerides go DOWN
7. HDL goes UP
8. Insulin Resistance goes DOWN
9. Insulin Sensitivity goes UP
10. WE are HAPPIER and HEALHIER!

STOP the PRESS this last section just said it all. **Happier** and **Healthier**, what is that worth? If you got it here, what did this book cost? Tell a friend **NOW!**

ATP Training includes a decrease in: Oxygen (O_2) cost and ventilation, given the same power output. We become more efficient, better gas mileage so to speak, improved strength to weight ratio, or as quantified in cycling- more Power in terms of watts per kilo (W/kg)

- The result is we have the capacity to sustain greater and greater intensities of movement- aerobically- funded by fat.

We would like to suggest that Power, Speed or Pace @FFA-ATP and LBP are better indicators of aerobic endurance than VO_2 max, as AT can change without improvement to VO_2 max. Performance improves and isn't that the whole point of study and activity? At M360 we will define and document your average wattage per kilo at 70%- FFA, 80% ATP and 85% LBP for 2', 4', 6', 10', 20 and 60'.

A Case for Aerobic Exercise and Lipid Panel

M360 Aerobic exercise involves cardiorespiratory endurance exercises and 50/70 resistance training. Increasing Power/Strength to Weight Ratio can improve health.

- Studies involving ATP aerobic exercise reported that HDL cholesterol, increased by 4.6 % whilst triglyceride levels fell by 3.7 % over a 8 week period.
- Pinpointing our intensity, duration and frequency is critical to the optimization of your metabolic health.

Remember that old saying: "it is not what you do, but rather **HOW** you do it"

Duration vs. Intensity and Lipid Panel

M360 suggests that HDL cholesterol is the lipid most likely to improve as the result of the execution - of all 4-sections of this book, specifically with section 3 on physical activity/exercise. Research documents that aerobic exercise is directly linked to an increase in **HDL.**

Research also proves that:

**Our lipid profiles are best improved by, our
Volume of Training, as opposed to our Intensity!**

Many studies indicate, that the key to reduction in fat mass- is exercise duration- there is a direct relationship between body fat reduction and prolonged exercise.

- Evidence is clear that moderate-intensity exercise, like **M360 Clinical Fitness** is critical to increasing our HDL cholesterol.
- Moderate intensity for longer durations of activity has a greater impact on the reduction of atherogenesis/atherosclerosis (scarring of endothelial wall tissue followed by plaque and fat accumulation). For this reason our morning sessions at M360 are 90 minutes in duration as opposed to most programs running 45 minutes.

Resistance Training loads and Lipid Panel

When it comes to resistance training, increases in HDL cholesterol were significantly greater following a regime of repetitions by body part done at 50 % 1 Rep max and 70 % 1 Rep Max than following 110 % 1 Rep Max.

Again- evidence based "MODERATION" wins the Gold!

Many studies have proven that high intensity resistance training **DID NOT** have the same benefit as superior- **moderate-intensity resistance training. Moderate resistance training done in greater volume had a better effect on metabolic health than that of high intensity.**

Combined Functional Circuit Training

Aerobic exercise and resistance training done in various functional modes, circuits of intensity, duration, and frequency did a better job of improving our panel of biomarkers that monitors our success- than just straight biking or lifting.

As a starting point: People who are new to exercise- should be prescribed prolonged- low to moderate-intensity, aerobic exercise (45%-70% mhr).

Example would be to build up the ability to walk 30-60-then 90 minutes rather than to try and jog the same durations. Lower intensities, done longer in duration, executed more frequently till the metabolism and body composition adjust.

Functional circuit training- with variable resistance and movement should be done in a predominantly aerobic state (<85% mhr), with increased duration- before increased intensity.

- Lower-intensity exercise (<85 % 1 RM) is more effective toward metabolic health and fat adaption than higher-intensity exercise (>85% % 1 RM).

- Moderate Aerobic Intensity- Activities (<85%) done in circuits with resistance training will improve our **M360** Biomarker targets of:
  - Lower hs-CRP
  - Lower Triglycerides
  - Higher HDL
  - Better Insulin sensitivity/Less Insulin resistance (Better I/R Score)

Increase Volume at ATP (Aerobic Transition Point)

Time spent doing aerobic exercise is linked to an increase in HDL cholesterol levels within our M360 tested NMR profile.

M360 aerobic resistance training objectives should be to:

- Increased number of reps and sets, before increasing weight lifted. This formula has a greater impact upon the lipid profile than:
- High intensity (high weight - low-repetition training).

ANS and Anaerobic Threshold Activity

Intensity of exercise drives our *autonomic nervous system* (ANS) and manages the balance between sympathetic (up) and parasympathetic (down) states. The variability of our heart beat in terms of beat-to-beat interval quality and rhythm is a reflection of stress during large muscle mass, dynamic exercise sessions like: cycling, paddling, and swimming, walking and running. This is our Clinical lab and our therapy to measure, manipulate and modify stress, upward for metabolic stimulus- as well as downward for metabolic recovery.

At the end of the day we are practicing the induction and reduction of stress. As we learn how to control and manipulate our autonomic nervous system up and down- we also learn how to; increase and decrease our inflammation and oxidation.

M360 utilizes ATP training (Aerobic Transition Point Training)

The most significant physiological variable in endurance sports
Is the Metabolic Transition Point from Aerobic to Anaerobic

Scientists have explained the term in various ways like:

- Lactate Threshold
- Ventilatory Anaerobic Threshold
- Onset of Blood Lactate Accumulation (OBLA)
- Onset of Plasma Lactate Accumulation
- Heart Rate Deflection Point
- Maximum Lactate Steady State and
- Lactate Balance Point (LBP)

Each one of these modalities is a reflection of metabolic activity and human performance. People with the greatest genetic ability to uptake and utilize oxygen still need the right intensity and duration of training to achieve optimal human performance.

Even the greatest Olympic athletes need to develop more power-speed or pace performance at sub maximal levels and constantly be improving performance efficiency specific to the activity they are pursuing

Our anaerobic threshold is just a tick above what we consider our maximum aerobic capacity or VO2 max. The key to smart training is to use this reference point of metabolic transition to our benefit by training right up to the **Aerobic Capacity** or just at the onset of anaerobic intensity.

It is here at this metabolic sweet spot- where we start rapidly accumulating extra lactate in the 2-4 mmol range that we want to start spending some time. **Remember:** the purpose of this level of training is to improve/

expand our aerobic capacity and become more efficient at utilizing oxygen to create energy. The more efficiently we do this the less ROS-Inflammation and Oxidative Stress we will produce. We not only train athletes for winning, we train everyday humans for optimal metabolic health.

There is a power – pace- speed/heart rate relationship with these finely tuned metabolic capacities or thresholds. By correlating real values of Speed, Pace, Power (workload) output against **Metabolic Cost** referenced by percentage of max heart rate (mhr) we can pinpoint the value of our **M360** session without doing cardio pulmonary gas exchange testing (CPET). We call this sweet spot Aerobic Transition Point or ATP Training. There must be little to **NO** metabolic acidosis.

Anaerobic Threshold (LBP) Aerobic Ceiling (ATP) & Fat Threshold (FFA)

At **M360** we do incremental sessions we call "**Power Ramps**" targeting certain our recognized metabolic thresholds, and here is what we observe:

1. Our first **Metabolic Zone of Interest** we will master is maximum **Free Fatty Acid** utilization. We call this zone **FFA** for short, and it generally correlates with our aerobic intensities of 50%-75% of our maximum heart rate capability.

This metabolic correlation to cardio output is our Peak Fat BURNING level as a percentage of total energy produced during the activity.

During a power ramp (gradual increase in wattage/speed/pace) this may come around 65%-75% of maximum functional threshold power for the tested duration (4'-20'-60')-and around 70-75% of MHR as the Upper limit of this FFA training intensity.

Using a 20' session I do, the higher our 20 minute average power-versus- our average heart rate, the better off we will be; in terms of our GOAL- **Metabolic Efficiency** relative to athletic performance, life and baseline health goal of producing less ROS and Oxidative Stress.

Example of a 20' FFA session you will see in a few pages:

- At this writing I can sustain 200 watts for 20 minutes- which is 74% of my maximum 270 wattage average for a 20 minute test of my maximum 20' functional power. (200w is 74% of 270w)
- I can do this at a 20' average heart rate cost (fractionalization of max Vo2) of 73% of my max heart rate (166bpm x.73 =121bpm). In my case I can produce slightly **MORE** Submaximal Power to heart rate cost (cardio pulmonary cost) as a percentage of maximum. These are our M360 Reference Points and they level the playing field for ALL of us, especially as you start breaking it down into watts per kilo (w/kg). We will do that in class at a more advanced point.
- This is what separates M360 Clinical Fitness from other programs, we are factual, and evidence based "FUN" exercise done in a small group- against real "Measurable Markers" of health and performance. (CRP-HDL-Triglycerides-Insulin Resistance-PERR-Metabolic Power @ Living Thresholds)
- The goal of these **"Power Ramp"** sessions is to dramatically improve our metabolic capacity to utilize fat substrate to fuel higher and higher workloads, be it in life, or in athletics.
- People with lower metabolic fitness will achieve higher heart rates (metabolic cost) at lower and lower power outputs (workload).

Example: This person would have lower power outputs as a percentage of maximum 20' minute functional power vs. their heart rate cost. At a sample of 73% of max heart rate they may only produce 65% of max

20' minute power. Doesn't sound like a lot, but for endurance athletes and humans (who are endurance athletes by nature just to survive) it hits us where we **LIVE!** Remember we DO **Nothing** and **Too** much really well. The problem we this fact is that we live -metabolically "IN the MIDDLE". This is what gets **LOST** in all the programs out there, even at the level of the Olympic Training Center!

To Conclude FFA:

In a gas exchange CPET test we would see this in Brilliant Colors: of Green, Orange, Blue and Red, please take a minute to go online -paste this link in and see the short video of an actual test I did with Cortex. https://www.metafit.life/feed/cpet-cardio-pulmonary-exercise-testing

You can also-s just go to www.metafit.life and you will find it under blogs. You will see that Fat Utilization peaks out as the Power Ramp goes up. It is our power at this point where fat as a substrate for ATP energy goes down to **ZERO** and Glycogen shoots up. This point of intersection (+) is the upper threshold of our **M360** FFA training sessions. **M360** will maximize your ability to live as a healthy active human or as an Olympic athlete. This is a critical Metabolic Zone for ALL of us; one that is almost always gets overlooked. This is where we should spend over 50% of our physical activity and exercise time- not in metabolic acidosis at some crazy xfit scam or overzealous mindless spinning session. This metabolic zone is where we live! This metabolic zone is where we learn to become Fat Adapted and as you will see in more of the book a great place to metabolically manipulate with time restricted eating (TRE) and intermittent fasting (IF).

https://www.metafit.life/feed/cpet-cardio-pulmonary-exercise-testing

2. Our second (2nd) **Metabolic Zone of Interest** we will master is maximum output at our **Aerobic Transition Point**. We call this zone **ATP** for short, and it generally correlates with aerobic intensities of 70%-80% of our maximum heart rate capability.

This metabolic correlation to cardio output represents the upper limits of our Aerobic Capacity, or maximum capacity to up load and utilize oxygen with little to **NO** excessive lactate build up.

During a power ramp I did recently at ***Stages Performance*** office in Boulder Colorado I was able to do 20' at an average of 260 watts or 96% of my max tested 20' ftp output of 270w. I did this at an average cardio pulmonary output of 132 beats per minute (bpm) which is 80% of my max 166bpm

This is great news is this reflects a very strong aerobic capacity for a 60 year old man. I can produce 96% of my total power at just 80% of my maximum cardio output- keeping my metabolic cost very low. This is my Power@ATP.

What is YOUR power at ATP? Join me and let's improve it!

In life this is partially **WHY** my hs-CRP is only .4, as this metabolic efficiency produces less ROS and more endogenous anti-inflammatory response to stress in daily life.

This is what I want for YOU to gain from M360! Metabolic Nirvana

3. Our third (3ʳᵈ) and final M360- **Metabolic Zone of Interest** we will master is our maximum output at Lactate Balance Point (LBP). We call this LBP for short, and it generally correlates with anaerobic intensities of 80%-90% of our maximum heart rate capability. We will spend less than 10% of our time here, more like 5%-7% of total training time, unless you are ramping up to compete in a special event.

This metabolic correlation to cardio output represents our maximum workload capacity just below or at Onset of Blood Lactate Accumulation (OBLA) exceeding 4mmol/L. I cannot tell you how many times I have tested this threshold with a blood lactate monitor- preparing for the

2008 Olympic Trials of Sprint Paddling, in an effort to raise my Power-Speed and Pace at OBLA, sometimes referred to as Power@Lactate Threshold (P@LT).

What is your POWER output at LBP and how long can you sustain it?

I do not spend much time here so I cannot spend a lot of time here writing, nor is it needed. To reference my latest effort at this level it was a Zwift Race over 20 minutes where I did my current 20' ftp of 270w. By the way this is only in the 3.4 w/kg area. Not bad for a 60 year old man, but my real goal is to keep this into my 70's and 80's. **Where are YOU and WHERE will we be in 10 years…20 years?**

Our unhealthy society of **Nothing** and **Too Much**, spends **TOO Much Time** here -not knowing the harm they are doing. It's a weird dynamic when you are in my shoes as a performance facilitator/fitness entrepreneur- people want to overdo it, and whip them into a frenzy of sweat to justify the expense and feel like they got their monies worth! Wouldn't it be better to train smart, not over-train and burn yourself out? Wouldn't it be better to set our program accountable to measurable/documentable improvement?

This is **WHY M360** only uses **3** levels of intensity to achieve our metabolic goals. FFA- ATP up to LBP. We are training to optimize our metabolic fitness for life.

M360 pedagogy allows us to do this and to document the process along with biomarker improvement. Think of our 3rd level of intensity (LBP) as being a point of balance that we exercise up to and tap against in repetition, or in tempo just below or at this fine **Metabolic Balance Point**. Remember our key is **Stimulate- not Destroy** our metabolism to optimize function in a sustainable fashion.

Do you know where this shift occurs in your own cardiorespiratory training?

Remember: We tend to do **NOTHING** or **TOO** much, whilst the real benefits of physical activity occur in between, where we really live. What we can now pinpoint with **M360** is the right mixture of Exercise and Activity on a weekly basis to- improve our:

- Fat metabolism
- Reduce metabolic acidosis
- Expand Aerobic Capacity and improve our health?

Finding the Sweet spot of ANS activation and Blood Chemistry

The 1st century Roman philosopher Marcus Cicero declared:

"Never go to excess, but let moderation be your guide."

The wisdom of this philosophy should be applied to all aspects of our lifestyle: eating, drinking, sleeping, working, playing — and exercising!

Ventilation Threshold (Breathing Rate)

As exercise intensity increases- just like our blood lactate suddenly SPIKES (2-4 mmol) and goes up, our rate of breathing also SPIKES (24-42 bpm) and does the same thing, this is often referred to as our ventilatory threshold. I threw this in so you will know the term when I mention it in a podcast or in a session.

Delivery of O2 is Critical for Fat Adaption and Exercise Intensity

Our max VO$_2$ is limited by the ability of our cardiorespiratory system to **"uptake and utilize oxygen"** by the active muscles specific to the activity we are performing.

How well do you Uptake and Utilize Oxygen? Want to improve it?

Relationship between Percent HR Max and Percent VO2 Max

As aerobes on the oxygen dependent planet earth, our capacity to perform aerobic physical activity and exercise is a critical component of our health and ROS/Inflammation management. Proper FFA and ATP- Aerobic activity rarely gets the appropriate emphasis it deserves in regard to cardiopulmonary improvements.

The M360 Principle of Nothing or Too Much!

"Cardio Gym Rats" climb onto aerobic ergo meters and start grinding away without ever taking into account any **Metabolic Training Zone** of any Duration, Intensity or Frequency in which they could or should be working to achieve metabolic health.

- It is common place in any gym to see cardio rats reading the paper while riding or watching the television. Time void of any-specific purpose- with little to no cardiovascular benefit?
- The flip side is former athletes (jocks), or wannabe's athletes stuck in this ridiculous endless loop of: **"Getting Back Into Shape"** inaccurately recalling former training volume/intensity of the good ole days- while attempting far too highly intense activities, only to quit, suffer injury, burnout gain weight and then do it all over again next January. Don't be this poor lost soul! This is the profile of most X fitters and it is ridiculous. Just check their CRP and you will know.

NOTE: Don't be Ridiculous!

To make the most of each exercise session or physical activity; you should train smart in an appropriate and systematic, evidence based manner. Unlike resistance training where you perform endless repetitions to failure or lift to a designated number, why not base your lifts on a percentage of maximum force output? Use reference point training and pinpoint your efforts rather than going at it blind and getting injured.

Why not use evidence based percentage% of your 1-Rep Max.?

Our capacity to move is **ALWAYS** based on a relative percentage of our maximal oxygen consumption. Why not lift weights and perform exercises in a fun and feel good format by utilizing **M360 Reference Point Training (RPT)?**

Resistance training is simple, pick your body part, and get an idea of your 1 rep max and alternate 2-3 days a week doing repetition of **50%-70%** of your 1- Rep max. With RPT when your 1- rep max goes up- with an occasional test, so do the parameters of your future training sessions.

The same principle is true of building your **AEROBIC CAPACITY** at transition point to anaerobic. In this case it is not weight lifted but Power, Speed or Pace produced at 3 simple intensity levels. Power @, Speed @or Pace @ FFA, ATP and LBP, obviously the goal would be to improve the workload at same metabolic expense or METABOLIC COST!

	FFA	ATP	LBP
% VO2Max	40% -50%	51% - 66%	66% - 82%
HR %max	45%-70%	70% - 80%	80% - 90%

Example: I just took a break from writing and did 4 – 20' minute segments on my Zwift/Cyclops Hammer Smart trainer and was able to do:

1. **170** watt avg. for 20' @ avg. of 111 bpm –or- **67%** of my max **166** bpm heart rate. **NOTE***I will be 60 in a few months and weigh 180 pounds or 81.6 kilo with a currently tested 1-hour FTP of 250 watts or 3.06 w/kg.
    a. My strength to weight ratio (STWR) at **67%** of my Max Heart Rate (MHR) is **2.08** watts per Kilo.
    b. **>Bullet Point: what will my 20'- 67% STWR be in 10 years @ 70 yrs old?**

2. **On the second one I did: 180** watt avg. for 20' @ 114 bpm avg. −or- **68%** of my mhr.
   a. My **STWR** @ 68% was **2.2** w/kg of my MHR.
   b. > **Bullet Point: What will my 20' -68% STWR be @ 80 years old?**
3. **On the 3rd one I did: 190** watt avg. for 20' @ 115 bpm avg. −or- **69.2%** of my mhr.
   a. My **STWR** @ 69% was **2.32** w/kg of my MHR.
   b. > **Bullet Point: What will my 20' -69% STWR be @ 80 years old?**
4. **On the 4th one I did: 200** watt avg. for 20' @ 122 bpm avg. −or- **73%** of my mhr.
   a. My **STWR** @ 73% was **2.45** w/kg of my MHR.
   b. > **Bullet Point: What will my 20' -73% STWR be @ 80 years old?**

Today my FFA capacity is between 190 w and 200w for 20'.

- I want you to notice how there was as little jump in Cardio (Heart Rate) Cost from 190 watts to 200 watts.
- This clearly points out a bit of a **Metabolic Threshold** or **Inflection point**. A potential **Transition Point** from our zone of **FFA** to our zone of **ATP**,
- With this we identified as a prime FFA/ATP zone I should be TARGETING- POWER gains @ 73-75% over 20 minutes. This is my FFA/ATP Sweet spot!

I hope this didn't run you too far off in the weeds, but as you can see these metrics are very concrete standards of our **POWER- VITALITY** and **FUNCTION** in **LIFE!**

The goal of **M360 Clinical Fitness** and **OUR** health is to get us, and keep us **POWERFUL** as long as possible, and then slow your rate of decline- from powerful to deceased with **NO FUNCTION**, as much as possible.

The solution to this scenario is for us to optimize, and personalize all 4-sections of this book. Start here and build on what I have pulled together. I know personally that all of this works. The metrics in each section keep me excited about each and every day of life. My intent is that you join me in the journey, and get excited over being:

- **Metabolically Fit for Life.**

For more on how we define training zones to best reflect utilization of food energy: Visit our website at https://www.metafit.life/feed/cpet-cardio-pulmonary-exercise-testing

Training Intensity and Metabolic Pathway Stress Response (ANS/HRV)

When we exercise at our **M360 ATP** level, between 70%-80% of our max heart rate we have a much higher use of fat and a slower depletion of muscle glycogen storage than when we exercise at or above AT level.

This aerobic transition point (ATP) intensity is a prime metabolic training zone for tempo sessions 20'-90' minutes in duration. It is here, with a great base of FFA that we will improve our metabolic function for life, with the least amount of oxidative stress or damage.

- When we keep the intensity of our sessions in a low to moderate range we keep our fat metabolism activated, and our sugar metabolism down-regulated.
- This dynamic dramatically flip-flops when our intensity goes above this transition point and our Sugar/Carbohydrate metabolism takes over and Fat Utilization goes to **ZERO**. Our training opportunity is lost!

Training just below –or- at anaerobic threshold level- what we call **"LBP Training"** results in:

- **Improved Muscle Structure**
- **Improved Capilarization**
- **Improved Fat Substrate utilization** (fat adaption)

Our benefits here should include:

- A decrease in our oxygen (O_2) cost per unit of ventilation
- Lower accumulations of lactate
- Less depletion of glycogen at a given point of power output, thus preserving our precious glycogen stores for maximal efforts called upon during emergencies as fight or flight or at the end of a race to win!

The end result is we improve! We get stronger; we can sustain more power longer and stay aerobic in a fat burning mode. We become increasingly metabolically efficient which improve our ability to reduce inflammation and oxidation. Again- metabolically fit for life!

Real Fitness is Sustainable Sub Maximal Metabolic Performance

Our performance capacity at each of our M360 training levels of: FFA, ATP and LBP are a better indicator of our aerobic endurance capacity than VO_2 max, as they all can be improved with proper training- without changes in VO_2 max.

This is where we live- is it not?

I already made the comment that we as humans do two things really well, nothing and too much. We do not live at either end; we live metabolically in the middle. Life is a journey of **SUSTAINED** effort and to get through it in flying colors we need to perform at 3 levels in the middle **FFA- ATP** and **LBP.** It all comes down improving our **USE of OXYGEN** (O_2) and our **UTILIZATION of FAT!** Everything we do at **M360** will be pointing at perfecting our metabolic health at every level we can access it!

Aerobic training improves our performance potential at peak FFA- at peak- ATP and at peak- Lactate Balance Point (LBP), without an increase in VO_2 max. Another fact based reason **WHY -M360** will only focus on the first 3 intensities of metabolic training (FFA-ATP-LBP).

Metabolically this is where we live, work, play, and perform!

Done correctly, exercise should produce just enough stimulation to be temporarily pro-inflammatory and increase oxidative stress in the **short term**; but create long term adaptations and benefits that will strengthen our ability to reduce our own personal **endogenous** - inflammatory reaction, while lowering oxidative stress- by optimizing our own **endogenous** antioxidant system- long term. To do this **M360 Clinical Fitness** recognizes that it is critical to be able to adjust, and fine tune- the following factors up and down accordingly: Modern technology helps us to pinpoint and deliver:

- **Intensity, Duration, Frequency to muscle mass involved in activity**

When we target specific physical stimulus- as we do at **M360**, utilizing personal metrics, we can pinpoint metabolic adaptations, and increase our metabolic resistance to ROS- which results in a marked increase in our endogenous antioxidant defense systems.

Along with this improved metabolic defense, we are able to document our power per kilogram gains, our Recovery/HRV, our CRP, our Insulin Sensitivity, our HDL and our Triglyceride level.

Our metabolic fitness journey is no longer the mystery it once was; we can pinpoint and fine tune our efforts and document our results. As a sick society, it is time to come out of the cave, and use our brains to optimize our metabolic function. Our future is **NOT** another burpee, or a deeper squat, it is a dramatically improved aerobic capacity and **FAT ADAPTATED METABOLISM.**

M360 endurance training –fine tuned at the proper intensity and duration- leads to physiological adaptations that include -activation of mitochondrial:

- **Biogenesis** – Generation of new cells, new mitochondria, New Life!
- **Fiber type transformation** – Improved Oxidative Capacity in muscle
- **Angiogenesis** – Creation of New Blood Vessels

These are the gains we are looking for, again-not another burpee or a deeper squat and blown out knees.

Almost sounds like a miracle or fountain of youth when you think about it. **M360** aerobic training stimulates:

- Strength to weight ratio -human muscle growth
- Fat Metabolism- aerobic capacity
- General resistance to fatigue- Stamina
- Increased endogenous anti-inflammatory capacity-OS defense
- Reduced Oxidative Stress and ROS
- Dramatically reduced proclivity toward Chronic Disease

Aerobic Transition Point (ATP) training with a strong FFA (Fat Adapted) base will stimulate short term- moderate production of free radicals; however this has been proven to be followed by an activation of the antioxidant defense system. This is much like Dr. Vigils super compensation model defined at our website: www.metafit.life under blogs. We train and break down or actually lose fitness (catabolic), but done correctly we adapt and recover and get stronger (anabolic) over the long term. Remember the MOST important PART of your Day is? _____

Research suggests that getting our intensity, duration and frequencey correct- is the key to our lifestyle component of EXERCISE contributing to the reduction of our inflammation and oxidative stress markers.

Our metabolic performance at our own personal Aerobic to Anaerobic transition point is the most important physiological parameters, in life and endurance sports. Keep in mind- life itself- is an endurance sport!

M360 Metabolic Transition points to focus on are:

Above I clearly stated from a test taken today- my power (avg. watt) at transition from **FFA-ATP** was right around **200 watts** for a **20'minute test**. As we identify these markers our training gains in accuracy. We can pinpoint and target progressive metabolic improvements with minimal chance for overtraining.

- **45%-70% mhr (FFA)** give or take 5% by fitness level.
  - **Example:** when we are in poor fitness Maximum Power at FFA may come at just 65% of MHR whilst when we are highly fit, it may come at 75% of MHR. I use 70% as a middle ground average. Our goal is to stay FFA/Aerobic as long as possible.
- **70%-80% mhr (ATP)** give or take 5% by fitness level
  - **Example:** when we are in poor fitness Maximum Power at ATP may come at just 75% of MHR whilst when we are highly fit, it may come at 85% of MHR. I use 80% as a middle ground average. Our goal is to stay Aerobic as long as possible before transitioning into an Anaerobic Metabolic State
- **80%- 90% mhr (LBP)** give or take 5% by fitness level
  - **Example:** when we are in poor fitness Maximum Power at LBP may come at just 85% of MHR whilst when we are

highly fit, it may come at 95% of MHR. I use 90% as a middle ground average. Our goal is to keep our power UP an our Onset Of Blood Lactate Accumulation DOWN as long as possible before hitting a state of Metabolic Acidosis. This is a zone we will use sparingly and when we do we will just tap on it then recover and tap on it again done in and intermittent interval structure.

- **50%-70% of 1 rep max resistance training**
  - ○ Reference is a beautiful word! We utilize reference point training (RPT) as it keeps us healthy, strong and moving forward. **Example** here is a bench press for our chest. Let's say your 1 rep max (1 maximal effort) is 100 pounds. Based on this test we would have you lift 50 pound reps on a 50% day- done in the 10-14 rep range and 70 pound reps on a 70% day- done in the 6-8 rep range. This formula will reduce stress, and injury, but stimulated growth, and strength. When your #reps at each reference point- go up, I guarantee you 1 rep max will follow, and the entire formula shift **UPWARD** when **YOU** are **READY**, not when some clown yelling at you says it is time to increase the weight.
- **Combination Circuit Training**
  - ○ Simple 50% lifts and combination exercises done on and off our Smart Trainers.

Million Dollar Question

As we age is our **Functional Capacity** at each one of these reference points going- **UP** or **DOWN?**

You have the <u>POWER</u> to modify the answer today!

Exercise Activities improved by Intermittent Fasting (See Podcasts)

Fasting promotes catabolism- along with the cleaning up of cellular damage. *Autophagy* is the process of cleaning up and recycling our cellular health. Periods of fasting and catabolism clean up our cells and rejuvenate our metabolism, setting the stage- for periods of eating and rebuilding (Anabolism). Together there is a **BALANCE** that optimizes our metabolic health and capacity to perform.

That's where our **M360** program comes into play- by providing just enough exercise stimuli to promote the catabolic process- followed by enough recovery to prompt regeneration of cells.

We will also dive into Time Restricted Eating (TRE) - (a form of Intermittent Fasting) that works around our physical and mental training (motivation/recovery) to optimize our cellular efficiency and with it metabolic fitness.

But that's only the first step...

The second step is to arrest the catabolic process in our muscle and promote recovery. For this promotion we need to feed our muscle need, with fast assimilating protein right after exercise. **Feed the Need!**

Quality whey protein is our best bet.

Right after exercise there is a two hour period called **"WINDOW of OPPORTUNITY"** in which our muscle tissue is most receptive to assimilate protein and nutrients directed at- recovery and growth. To best take advantage of this opportunity we must feed our muscle mass during this window- with fast assimilated quality protein such as a quality whey protein. During this window- slow assimilating proteins won't do the job. Meat, poultry and fish are too slow assimilating and therefore will not fit post exercise recovery, anabolic opportunity. Whey protein powder time!!!

Physical activities in an Un-Fed State

- Exercising in and **UN-FED** calorie restricted state has many health and performance benefits.
- Exercising in an **UN-FED** fasted state stimulates our sympathetic nervous system (SNS) and activates our capacity to burn fat.

Our body's fat burning processes are controlled by our Sympathetic Nervous System (SNS), which is activated by physical activity and by lack of food. Research points out that fasting can trigger a dramatic increase in human growth hormone (HGH). When I say dramatic I mean dramatic, some studies throw around numbers like a 1,300% increase in women and 2,000% increase in men. Keep in mind this is a good thing, these are not exogenous increases, these are the endogenous workings of a healthy metabolism taking care of itself to repair, rebuild and renew cellular tissue.

Remember my experience with Dr. Leslie Shooter at the Olympic Training Center when she said: "Tim, it is all a matter of Load and Recover". This is it in a nutshell, break it down without permanent damage, clean it out and rebuild it. This process basically keeps us cellularly- **NEW** (young).

A *combination* of exercising and fasting, when done correctly- will maximize the metabolic impact to utilize fat and glycogen for energy.

- Training on an empty stomach effectively forces our body to burn fat.

I want **YOU** to get excited, because it is my guess that you are **NOT** currently **FAT ADAPTED**, meaning your metabolism is not real good at burning **FAT** for **FUEL**. You are in for a **DRAMATICALLY-IMPROVED** way to live. One that is much more energy efficient, meaning you will have a dramatic increase in energy to use on building healthy lean muscle mass and literally melting down fat storage to be utilized as high octane **ENERGY**, done in a healthy sustainable fashion.

NOTE: we have discussed oxidative stress (OS), which is created during catabolic periods, in a negative light, and yes when it is *chronic* it can lead to chronic disease. But *acute* oxidative stress, which occurs during exercise or periodic fasting, will actually benefit our muscle tissue when we allow our **BODY** and **MIND** to **RECOVER** properly. Once again it is a matter of **Load** and **Recover**. The key to success is being able to adequately recovery from specific targeted stress. This is what separates our program from others!

Intermittent Fasting for General Health and Longevity

Intermittent fasting (IF) has a beneficial effect on our health and longevity. Keep in mind that everything we do, are required to do, or **choose** to do- has an effect on our metabolism. The type of exercise and timing of nutrients to support and feed the needs of -**what we do**- is a blank canvas we have control over. Intermittent fasting is a choice, but it is just one of a number of tools we have control over to optimize our metabolic health.

Studies have confirmed that fasting will assist our metabolic function by:

- Optimizing our insulin sensitivity (reducing our I/R score) which will assist our cells in counteracting our rate of aging, as well as assisting us in the regeneration and repair of muscle tissue.
- The key target of **M360** is to normalize our insulin sensitivity, and reduce inflammation/oxidation that leads to nearly **ALL** chronic disease.
- Normalize "Our hunger hormone" or ghrelin levels
- Fasting is proven to elevate human growth hormone (HGH) levels which are important to our health, fitness and ability to slow the aging process.

- Lower triglyceride levels
- Reduce inflammation and free radical damage (ROS)

Similar to calorie restriction (CR), Intermittent fasting (IF) can improve health and extend lifespan by:

- Decreasing our plasma insulin (lower I/R score)
- Decreasing our blood sugar concentrations
- Decreasing our blood pressure
- Decreasing our resting and functional heart rate
- Enhancing our immune function
- Reduced our body fat
- Increasing our Energy Level

Muscle Degradation and Premature Aging

Muscle tissue tends to degrade as we age, which quickly becomes a major factor in the decline of our bodily functions. **Atrophy** of our **Muscle Mass** is much more than just the loss of our muscle strength and size; atrophy left unchecked will lead to metabolic decline. We must take action, and take action **NOW** to arrest this decline, and even turn it around, and build it back up!

Muscle Mass goes beyond motion. Muscle mass is our largest source of energy production. Muscle mass keeps our metabolism humming along and is responsible for:

- Metabolic and Hormonal improvement or decline
- Obesity or Healthy lean composition.
- Diabetes or healthy blood sugar/fat balance
- Cardiovascular disease or Optimum CV function
- Enhanced cognitive function that keeps your body young, or a decline of cognitive function and premature aging

You are at a FORK in the ROAD. Right is Health, Left is Sickness and Misery, what direction are you going to GO?

Muscle atrophy leads to other major health issues you may want to consider.

Loss of Muscle Mass will Result in:

- **Loss of energy**
- **Excessive tendency to gain weight**
- **Vulnerability to disease**
- **Accelerated aging**

Muscle decline is a major factor in the epidemics of diabetes, obesity, and other related diseases.

Why does or Muscle Tissue Atrophy?

The short list includes:

- Nutritional abuse
- Insulin resistance
- Hormonal disorders
- Inflammatory disease
- Oxidative **STRESS**
- Muscle injury
- Dietary abuse
- Inactivity

Oxidative ROS Damage of Un-checked Free Radicals

As we now know, reactive oxygen species ROS, are toxic - they bind up and invade our body as they destroy our cells and damage our metabolism.

Our body defends us against these destructive particles with our own endogenous antioxidants such as- glutathione along with dietary antioxidants we get from the food we eat.

Are we getting these antioxidants?

Unless we proactively guard against these ROS concentrations they will overwhelm our body's defenses, destroy our cells- destroying cellular proteins, lipids, and eventually our DNA.

Accumulated of ROS leads to at least 3- detrimental changes:

- **Loss** of energy producing mitochondrial function
- **Loss** of fast neuro motor facilitation
- **Loss** of fast reacting muscle fibers and reduced mobility

Loss of Mitochondrial Function

- Oxidative damage in our mitochondria will promote the following:
  - **Chronic infections**
  - **Chronic inflammatory and chronic disease**
  - **Chemical toxicity and rancid fat**
  - **Excessive sugar or fructose intake**
  - **General mitochondrial impairment**

Are you a victim of your own program?

Overtraining from exercise programs that do not monitor and document the physiological effects of intensity duration and frequency are the biggest cause of mitochondrial damage. I see these crazy sessions of other programs from spin sessions to x-fit madness and I cringe at the damage they are causing in the name of health and human performance. It really is nonsense and an insult to our intelligence.

Not knowing why, when, or how to adjust the intensity, duration or frequency up or down is a blindness we no longer have to endure. **M360** is here to help you pinpoint the proper mixture of components that will improve **ALL** the **BIOMARKERS** we seek to optimize.

The <u>Train Wreck</u> of <u>Bad Nutrition</u> and <u>Bad Training</u>

Bad nutrition- with bad training liter today's **"Fitness Landscape"** with extremely destructive consequences that -over time- will lead to irreversible damage of our mitochondria along with total metabolic decline. **Are you X- Fitters, Grunting Gym Rats and Whoop-Whoop Go Girl Spinners listening?**

The consequences include:

- Impaired ability to utilize carbohydrates and **FAT** for **ENERGY**
- Insulin resistance
- Lower threshold for physical exercise
- Excessive weight gain
- Accelerated aging

How You Lose Fast Twitch Neuromuscular Capacity

Our neuromuscular system controls all of our physical movement. When we are over exposed to chronic - oxidative stress our neuromuscular schematic begins to deteriorate.

I have always made the analogy of a light switch, and a wire from the switch to a light bulb. Unless the wire communicates power from the switch to the bulb there is **NO LIGHT**. If we destroy our wiring, oxidize our nervous system- then we no light, there will be **NO** movement, or severely impaired movement. I have always referred to the training of this system and NMF training or Neuro Muscular Facilitation. At **M360** we do this with balls, bands, sticks and balance.

The guy who coined the phrase **"No Pain No Gain"** should be **LOCKED UP-** along with the Gal that said: **"I didn't get this way sleeping"...** SAY WHAT?

Resistance Training regardless of Age is Critical!

Our neuro-muscular system is subject to age-related damage, from a lack of stimulation, and years of abuse via poor diet/lifestyle. This damage is why we lose:

- **Power**
- **Speed**

As we age, if we choose to do **NOTHING** to maintain and increase muscle function, strength and mass then we will lose function of our neuro-motors and along with it the ability to execute daily functions to live a normal independent life. Why we do this to ourselves is beyond me.

I see guys my age retire and flop onto the couch, claiming independence from working. The sad reality is they just initiated a miserable ride of morbidity toward a miserable death!

Why not use the free time of retirement- to adopt the principles we are discussing here- and get in the Metabolic Shape of our Life!

OUR Immune System and Exercise

Moderate exercise has a protective effect on our immune system- whereas overly strenuous exercise - results in immune dysfunction. Again measured moderation is the key to a balanced and efficient metabolism that promotes optimum immunity.

Practical M360 Exercise Prescription

Our M360 Prescription to the general public is:-

1. Any new exercise or physical activity regime should start at a **low intensity** below 70% of maximum heart rate (MHR) with durations of 45 minutes to 1-hour.
2. Gradually adapting to a few segments a week –to reflect -**moderate intensity** at or less than 80% mhr (60% -65% VO_2max) with durations up to 60 minutes/session.
3. The final transition would be to allocate a few days a week for measured sessions up to and slightly above 85% mhr with durations up to and beyond 90 minutes, staying out of metabolic acidosis and taking into account adequate recovery, with the global assessment of recovery markers like:
   a. Resting heart rate (RHR) and heart rate variability (HRV).

A Case for Moderate Evidence Based Exercise

We have learned over the last 40 years that moderation is the key to metabolic success.

In my pursuit of breaking 4 minutes in the mile run and so many other competitions in my life- I have pushed the upper limits of intensity to the max, and have learned the value of moderation – measured – metabolically stimulating exercise and physical activity.

Moderate intensity exercise is the best and results in a **reduced stress hormone response**, which promotes a **favorable immune response**. It is absolutely crazy to me that exercise programs for the most part do not have any reference point in which to position the **"Individual"** amongst the **"Group"**.

Each individual has a unique metabolism. Our first goal of **M360** is to discover the unique parameters and limiting factors of each individual with the assistance of our unique monitoring technologies.

If the stimulus for gain is lifting a weight that it 50% or 70% of that individual's 1-rep maximum lift by body part, then we will know what that value is, and operate according to scale of RPT.

The objective of any program should be to provide just the right amount of **"Stimulus"** to produce a moderate metabolic action that brings a positive change to the metabolic systems of each individual. That may be 3 x 20 minutes of steady state ATP aerobic activity at 80% of your maximum power output, or it may be 2-hours of steady FFA at 50% of your max power output. Regardless of the content of the session, in or out of our facility, it will be **RELEVANT** and **SPECIFIC** to the **INDIVIDUAL** regardless of age, gender etcetera.

Exercise, Aging, Immunity and Inflammaging

Age-associated *senescence* and *immune deficiency* are at least partly responsible for the detrimental effects of old age. These unaltered effects of the "wear and tear" of age, gradually destroy our immune system, producing a low-grade inflammation referred to as **"inflammaging"**. As we age it is more and more and more important that we address inflammaging and realize what we are up against.

Our healthcare system must have a program of defense that integrates all 4 sections of our book and **M360** program: Lifestyle, Exercise, Nutrition and Stress Management to reduce and eliminate the debilitating effects of age.

It is my personal opinion that we do not have to suffer as we do, if we would just alter our mindset, and learn better ways to execute our 16 hour day.

Gradual loss of function is the most prominent downside of aging and it begins and ends at the cellular level. We are **ALL** up **AGAINST** the age-related loss of function that ultimately leaves us susceptible to many miserable conditions of:

- **Infection**
- **Autoimmune disorder**
- **Cancer**

M360 will always monitor Power- Vitality and Function (PVF) relative to the individual. Some portion of each session will always focus on keeping our power to weight, or strength to weight ratio at the very highest level- we possibly can, thus arresting the inevitable slide- to loss of function, and death.

Recent research is beginning to understand the specific connection between aging and lifestyle- (in particular, exercise and diet).

What this research is finding is that our mitochondria play a critical role in our process of aging. Research is beginning to understand how we can target and manipulate senescent cellular function. Manipulations that show promise in delaying the onset of many age-associated disorders include:

- **Caloric restriction** (CR)
- **Intermittent fasting** (IF) including (TRE)
- **Evidence Based Exercise** that targets stimulation of metabolism (EBE)

We have the enormous power of intervention on our side - if we would just adopt a mindset of learning new habits, behaviors and routines that can dramatically improve health longevity.

M360 seeks to target and support our mitochondria's impact on cellular aging with simple interventions into Lifestyle, Exercise, Diet and Stress mgmt.

Keep in mind this is a **WORK** in **PROGRESS**. Data is changing everyday as we become more informed on simple functional foods, exercise intensity, duration and frequency effects.

Our M360 premise is simple:

Why not use the latest science in conjunction with personal metrics and reference points to target and improve a select list of **KNOWN** issues that cut life short and reduce the quality of our existence. At the very base of it all, we are here to find Metabolic **HARMONY**, are we not?

What is cellular senescence?

Cellular senescence is centerpiece of aging. Senescence is one of the prime reasons that we age. Increasing numbers of our cells enter into a state known as senescence as we age. Senescent cells no longer divide or support the tissue they are part of; like problem children, they spew out a cocktail of harmful molecular signals that increase inflammation and oxidation that drives the aging process. They are basically gang banging thugs- hanging around- loitering, and disturbing normal cellular function.

Senescent cells can block important cellular processes, prevents stem cells from repairing damaged tissue promote the development of age-related diseases.

What if we can take simple steps in the course of our day to combat these destructive forces with a few simple alterations to our choice of Lifestyle -Exercise, Diet and Stress Management?

There are things we **CAN DO**, that show great potential to alter this situation.

Promising Steps we make part of our M360 program to combat senescence

- Exercise induced basal autophagy is a protective **"clean-up"** system that can result in stem cell regeneration.
- Autophagy is required for muscle stem cell balance and maintenance.
- Also called satellite cells (SCs) Muscle stem cells, are essential to muscle formation and regeneration.
- Physical exercise activates autophagy in skeletal muscles.
- Intermittent Fasting (IF) also has been proven to stimulate cellular autophagy and may assist in the removal or clearance of negative cellular senescence.

Research findings indicate that proper activation of autophagy is important for muscle homeostasis during physical activity. The intensity and duration of exercise stimulus can either improve or retard autophagy, yet another reason to utilize **SMART** training and personal metrics to measure and assure the proper Intensity- Duration and Frequency of our wellness program.

Lymphatic System <u>Moderate Aerobic Exercise</u> is best

The 1st century Roman philosopher Marcus Cicero declared:

"Never go to excess, but let moderation be your guide."

Again-these words should be applied toward all aspects of our life: eating, drinking, sleeping, playing, working, — and exercising!

Stimulating Sessions of **-Feel Good-** moderate intensity exercise are "immuno-enhancing" and can be used to effectively increase immune systems in patient/athletes.

Improvements in immunity due to regular exercise of moderate intensity are due to reductions in inflammation, alterations in the composition of "older" and "younger" immune cells, increased capacity to handle and manage psychological stress. Proper Exercise is indeed a powerful behavioral intervention that has the potential to improve immune and health outcomes at a variety of levels.

What is your <u>Balance Point</u> of Intensity, Duration and Frequency?

At what point does your Exercise or Lifestyle become Acidic or Toxic?

M360 Rx Summary of Effects:

Incremental improvements in **M360** activities and exercise routines **"in and out"** of our facility will target the improvement of all 10 of our Specific Biomarkers.

1. **FFA Training** - Fat Adaptation Training (FAT) will increased duration and power at highest possible yield of Adenosine Triphosphate from your Fat Metabolism (lipolysis). Power @ FFA

2. **Aerobic Transition Point** exercise (ATP Training) improves the capacity of muscle to oxidize fat (Beta Oxidation) Target Zone is **Power/Vitality** and **Function** @ 70-80% of MHR. Power @ ATP.

3. **FFA, ATP** and **LBP** training will target and increase **HDL-C** whilst lowering **Triglycerides**, and increasing **Insulin Sensitivity.**

4. **FFA, ATP & LBP** training will lower Blood Pressure to Optimum Levels.

5. **50-70 resistance training** will improve mobility, strength and cellular function. Keep in mind the value of maintaining even increasing lean mass as we age to preserve power and vitality vs. the loss of function.

6. **Improve resting Heart Rate Variability** (HRV)
7. **Improve the ability of Autonomic Nervous System** (ANS) to transition from Stimulated Sympathetic Mode to Recovering Parasympathetic Mode.
8. **Improve Active Recovery** from LBP to FFA 1 minute and 2 minute.
9. **FFA, ATP, LBP & 50/70** training will increase **Aerobic Power, Vitality** and **Function.**
10. Improve maximal **Post Exercise Recovery Rate** (PERR)
11. Improve Individual's **Strength to Weight Ratio** (STWR)
12. Lower overall **Cellular Inflammation**
13. Reduce overall **Cellular Oxidation**
14. **Improve Immune System** by stimulation of Lymphatic Schematic.
15. **Achieve optimal body compositions** of Lean Mass, Fat Mass and total Weight

What the HELL are POP Culture Xfit programs teaching our kids?

In our opinion and observation- pop cultural- boot camps and overly intense programs are doing more **HARM**- than good. The vast majority of the **"Fitness Programs"** that litter and confuse our health and wellness landscape, only generate more free radical stress and inflammation by being too difficult, intense and flat out wrong. Many have <u>**NO**</u> points of reference - to personalize the cornerstones of fitness:

- **Intensity**
- **Duration**
- **Frequency**

"Go Hard or Go Home" is about the most Ignorant Statement ever uttered!

1. **M360** takes the guesswork out of training and activity with the use of personal metrics.
2. Each individual has a unique variety of scientifically documented reference points that that they will work against.
3. Each workload is specific to the individual's metabolic capacity.
4. This approach will pinpoint the desired training effect of each modality of lifestyle we are targeting for overall metabolic fitness for life.

Protecting and Supporting Mitochondrial Performance

The beautiful fibers of our muscle mass contain both- enzymatic and nonenzymatic antioxidants- that work as a complex unit to regulate ROS (Reactive Oxygen Species).

- Within muscle fiber, antioxidants are strategically located throughout our cytoplasm and mitochondria.
- Enzymatic and nonenzymatic antioxidants live in extracellular and vascular space.
- Antioxidants protect muscle fibers from oxidative injury during periods of increased oxidant production- intense or prolonged exercise.

Chronic exposure to high levels of ROS (Free Radicals) is associated with the development of an increasing number of human diseases, such as:

- **Cardiovascular**
- **Metabolic**
- **Inflammatory and neurogenerative diseases**
- **Cancer**
- **Muscle atrophy**
- **Ageing process**

Help your body do- what your body was designed- to do!

Our magnificent body has several cellular antioxidant defense strategies to counterbalance ROS. These strategies include converting ROS into less active species and preventing the transformation of these less active molecules into ones with higher activity, scavenging ROS and minimizing the availability of pro-oxidants. The composition of antioxidant defenses differs from tissue to tissue and from cell-type to cell-type, but broadly, antioxidant defense systems can be classified into:

- **Endogenous** enzymatic and non-enzymatic antioxidants on the one side, and
- **Exogenous**, that is, dietary antioxidants on the other.

Examples of endogenously produced antioxidants are:

- **Glutathione** - Plays a crucial role in shielding our cells from endogenous and exogenous reactive oxygen and nitrogen species.
- **Bilirubin** – Works with glutathione to protect us from oxidation by ROS.

Oxygen is the base element of our aerobic life, we are aerobes yet oxygen is poisonous in many ways being linked to potentially dangerous oxidative damage. As aerobic organisms we must find new ways to survive these harmful effects. Our defense mechanism is our antioxidant system and we must **<u>SUPPORT</u>** it as much as possible with an intelligent lifestyle of:

- **Functional Foods**
- **Targeted Nutraceuticals**
- **Targeted Physical Activity and Meaningful Exercise**
- **Effective Stress Management and Meditation**

Segue into the Section 3 on Diet and Nutrition

In the next section we will explore what diet and nutrition really mean. Simply put- diet and nutrition support what we do. We call it **"Feeding the Need"**.

Our choice of lifestyle and activities must be supported by the foods we eat and the air we breathe. What we choose to eat and **WHY** is a serious question more folks should be exploring. Keep in mind this book is designed as a simple reference manual to our **M360** program. We will explore and define each topic over years of working together. We will explore modality after modality in a fun and entertaining way. This is **ALL** about **LIFE!** Embrace the **JOY** of **LIFE** and supporting our metabolism that is at work to bring us **LIFE** and Metabolic **ENERGY** to **LIVE.**

Preview into a few exogenous components of Anti-Inflammation and Oxidation

Our antioxidant defense systems work in a coordinated manner and are closely related to nutrition, key exogenous antioxidant substances we should find in our diet are:

- **Vitamin C**
- **Vitamin E**
- **Polyphenols** (e.g. flavonoids).
- **Sulforaphane**

Within the framework of this section, our focus is on vitamin C and E in the context of **M360** exercise sessions, as discussed below.

Exercise and Nutraceutical Supplementation to Reduce Oxidative Stress

Reactive Oxygen Species (ROS)/ Oxidative Stress (OS) produced during activity can prevent essential cellular/metabolic processes from taking place. To counter this we not only have physical activity/exercise sessions at **M360 we** are also lifestyle performance facilitators here to coach you on how to reduce and prevent this cellular damage and get the most out of our sessions.

In this situation we know that this increase in OS from our very own exercise program is:

1) Minimal because we only do 3 levels of intensity – low FFA, medium ATP and higher LBP with a rule to rarely go into intense metabolic acidosis.
2) Manageable because we can meet our antioxidative requirements with our balanced- Functional Whole Food diet rich in Nutraceuticals to defend us against oxidative stress and inflammation.

A Case for Vitamin C and Endurance Athletes

To further protect us against OS from exercise and OS in general it is suggested that we supplement our functional whole food diet with vitamin C and E. Vitamin C has been linked to protection us against atherogenesis via the prevention of LDL oxidation.

"Oxidation of LDL" is strongly associated with arterial plaque. Vitamin C (ascorbic acid or ascorbate) is also an essential micronutrient known to assist our:

- **Exercise Metabolism**
- **Exercise Immunology**

Vitamin C along with other antioxidants, help us to recover from mild muscle catabolism and inflammatory responses when they are at their highest after more intense sessions or with overall life stress in general.

Remember when it comes to life and training at any level it comes down to a cycle of:

"Load and Recover"!

Vitamin C is clearly linked to assisting our immune system in the process of recovery. In addition to vitamin C supplementation we need to get a variety of Functional Whole Food Nutraceutical antioxidants, vitamins, minerals etc in whole food combinations. **Example:** is Turmeric is better absorbed and bioavailable to our body as an antioxidant when it is consumed with the fat of an avocado served with salt and pepper, as is tomato with avocado and pepper to get the full effect of lycopene. We should all be encouraged to eat a diet rich in nutraceutical antioxidants from a broad variety of:

- Fresh Organic Vegetables and Fruit
- Fresh Organic Herbs and Spices
- Grass Fed Meats and Wild cold water fish
- Nuts and Seeds
- Good Oils and Fats (avocado, olives, avocado oil, olive oil, coconut oil)

To get more vitamin E, we can increase our intake of: avocados, nuts, seeds, asparagus, spinach, sunflower seeds, and good oils like avocado oil and olive oil.

High training volumes require more antioxidants, simply because we are creating more metabolic breakdown (catabolism). It is at this time we should consume more fresh organic fruit and vegetable juice like blueberry juice for polyphenols and beet juice for its vasodilatation and antioxidant qualities.

Vitamin E is for Endurance?

Vitamin E can play a key role in preventing atherosclerosis and other diseases associated with oxidative stress.

What are your current sources of Vitamin E? _____

I personally supplement vitamin E as it needed during periods of:

- Moderate to Intense training
- Long durations of endurance exercise lasting 4-8 hours
- During recovery periods after fasting or demanding training sessions.

The Ultimate Goal is to "<u>Feeding the Need</u>" as we call it

Our basic nutritional need is a reflection of what we do in terms of our "**CURRENT**" training load or demand.

Optimal bioavailability, of a variety (Matrix) of phytochemical and antioxidant compounds- derived from whole foods in the form of vegetables, fruits, and nuts should **NOT** be considered replaceable by supplementation.

Phytochemicals such as polyphenols are well recognized for their antioxidant properties; and should be consumed in whole food. **That said- during intense times of stress- minimal supplementation is reasonable.**

Supplementation may be critical to optimal performance?

Free radical (ROS) generation is greater when the intensity, duration and frequency of physical activity are increased. You are ultimately the judge on supplementation levels of Vitamin C and E.

Managing Markers of Human Performance and Health

C - Reactive protein (CRP) and Exercise

Research clearly dictates the value of physical activity and its role in preventing coronary heart disease, primarily for its role in lowing inflammation and oxidation.

Mode of Exercise and Activity vs. Inflammatory Response

- It is **NEVER** too late to take up exercise and lower our CRP/ inflammation levels and with it lower oxidative stress.
- Low to moderate intensity physical activity is the top correlate of CRP
- Increased cardiorespiratory fitness is strongly associated with a decrease in CRP levels.
- Exercise lowers inflammation as evidenced by reduced CRP levels. We would like to suggest that you get your hs-CRP Score below 1mg/L
- Moderate continuous and highly variable exercise training **modes** will reduce inflammation and suppresses CRP levels.

Documented modalities know to target lower CRP levels are:

- **Lower-carbohydrate diet** (developing a fat adapted metabolism)
- **Increased physical activity** (expanding duration and frequency)
- **Reduced inflammation** – lower oxidation and insulin resistance.

Exercise drives our "anti-inflammatory" state

- Physical activity can lower inflammation and improve endothelial function.
- Physical activity promotes nitric oxide availability that dilates and improves endothelial function.

M360 exercise training can reduce CRP

CRP is lowered with targeted low intensity high duration physical activity, moderate intensity exercise, and nutraceutical intervention along with stress mgmt techniques:

- Increasing insulin sensitivity
- Improving endothelial function
- Lowering Triglycerides
- Reducing body fat mass and body weight
- Raising HDL's

Chronic effects of moderate physical activity

- Moderate exercise promotes the release of pro-inflammatory cytokines that down regulate our sympathetic tonus and activate our parasympathetic nervous system that ultimately reduce oxidative stress.
- Moderate improves endothelial function by increasing levels of endothelium-derived nitric oxide. ***See Beet Juice and its nitric oxide value in the next section on Diet and Nutrition.***

Fat Adapted Metabolic Fitness and Efficiency

Converting to a diet rich in healthy fat- can lead to increased levels of fat oxidation/utilization during physical activity and exercise.

This change in diet supports lypolysis, and produces higher levels of plasma fatty acid (FA) during exercise. We call this FFA training or Free Fatty Acid utilization training. Lower intensity prolonged endurance training (90min +) done below 75% of max heart rate in conjunction with a fat-rich diet leads to measurable changes in our capacity to transport, recruit and oxidize fat as a ATP Fuel Substrate.

M360 Summary Bullet Points (Crib Notes)

- Choose a better structure of your waking 16 hour lifestyle
- Make time for "Effective" Exercise and Physical Activities
- Goal is to get you moving in the right direction to reduce Stress, Inflammation, Oxidation to eliminate conditions of chronic disease and poor performance.

- Improve your HRV
- Lower your hs-CRP
- Lower your Blood Pressure
- Increase your HDL
- Reduce your Triglycerides
- Improve your Insulin Sensitivity
- Improve your 1 minute and 1 minute recovery rates
- Improve your Strength to Weight Ratio
- Improve you Mobility and Balance/Self Awareness and Focus
- Lower your Fat Mass
- Improve your Fat Metabolism
- Reduce your Glycemic Load
- Increase your Lean Mass Relative to your Fat Mass
- Optimize your Body WEIGHT!

It should be quite obvious by now that we lack a program backed by science to help people recognize and implement a meaningful program to reduce conditions or biomarkers that will lead to Chronic Disease.

It is not just exercise, or activity or diet or stress management. Success comes when we target the cells and life giving mitochondria with all of the above in a CONCERT of SUPPORT rather than Sabotage!

It should be quite clear by now that our Lifestyles, Exercise Routines, Diet's and Lack of Stress Management have made us TOXIC.

We are Inflamed and decaying by excessive Oxidative Stress.

We CAN CHANGE and get on the RIGH TRACK, but we must do it in a sustainable way, so that the change takes for life. This is why we work in BLOCKS of 5 weeks, promoting your participation in multiple blocks per year until you DO NOT NEED US ANYMORE! You must take it upon yourself my friends.

Section #2 Summary:

Physical activity and exercise is an opportunity to move, and enjoy life. What we choose to do, and more importantly, **HOW** we choose to do it- is critical to our metabolic success.

As we age, and as our physical capability slides from **Powerful** to- **Vital** to- **Basic Function** we have more control of the slide- than ever thought possible.

WE have the opportunity to monitor biomarkers, and target our efforts- as we modify our performance outcomes. We no longer need to stumble around in the dark ages of all these ridiculous programs that never mention metabolic health and wellness. We can Target our metabolism- with a variety of modalities- done in a variety of Intensity, Duration and Frequency:

1. **Intensity**- "How Hard" we exert ourselves -relative to our maximum capacity for any given activity or exercise
2. **Duration**- "How Long" we exert ourselves –relative to our maximum capacity for any given activity or exercise.
3. **Frequency**- "How Often" we exert ourselves at some Intensity or Duration relative to our maximum capacity for any given activity or exercise.

Who here would argue that for the most part we humans, in particular- Americans do 2-things really well:

- **NOTHING & TOO MUCH**

We often do more harm than good with our programs. WELL that is all about to change- because we now have the technology and methodology for creative performance facilitators like me- to put together programs that provide "Evidence Based Programs" programs that are measurable, documentable and can prove- the improvement- of YOUR HEALTH!

We <u>CAN</u> lower our CRP

We <u>CAN</u> lower our Triglycerides

We <u>CAN</u> raise our HDL's

We <u>CAN</u> improve Insulin Sensitivity

We Can **PROVE** it! We can achieve it- with meaningful, targeted - **FEEL GOOD-** Exercise and Physical Activity.

We do **NOT** have to kill ourselves with tortuous routines; we simply need to stimulate various components of our metabolism, while having fun over a space of time.

We can target our own personal: optimal intensity, optimal duration, and optimal frequency within a variety of modalities- done in a sustainable fashion over the course of our life.

We get to **ENJOY** life! We can be healthier and perform better. We can enjoy **Metabolic Fitness for Life.**

SECTION #3

Diet

Nutrition

LIFESTYLE COMPONENT #3

Diet/Nutrition

Nutrition is what we derive from our diet. Diet is a misused word, misaligned with temporary fads and crazy marketing schemes, bombarding us with misinformation.

Diet Defined: is simply the food taken by a person or group of persons. **Nutrition** is the nutraceutical value of your diet in terms of how it affects your health and performance. Calories are **NOT** created equally. The critical point of our view on Nutrition and Diet is the answer to the question:

Does your diet provide the Nutrition that your Cells need to achieve?

- Optimal Health
- Wellness
- Higher Performance

Do you FEED the NEED!

This section will address **what** we eat and **how** it affects our body!

Does your Diet promote Inflammation and high levels of Oxidation?

A rise in chronic disease has brought a great deal of focus and spotlight on the science of free radical chemistry, ROS, silent inflammation and oxidative stress

What is a Free Radical?

Our bodies are under constant attack from oxidative stress (OS). Let's get a little technical, but stay with me, it is really very simple.

- Oxygen in the body splits into single atoms with unpaired electrons.
- Electrons like to be in pairs, so these atoms, called free radicals, scavenge the body to seek out other electrons so they can become a pair.
- This causes damage to DNA, cells, and proteins.

Free radicals are associated with human disease.

Free Radicals also have a link to our rate of aging, which is defined as a gradual accumulation of free-radical damage. My own mantra is:

"Show me Oxidation and Inflammation-and I will show you Conditions of Chronic Disease"!

Substances and Conditions that generate free radicals can be found in:

1. Foods we eat
2. Medicines we take
3. Air we breathe
4. Water we drink
5. Activities we do- have to do- or choose to do!

These substances and conditions include:

- Pharmaceuticals
- Chemical Toxins
- Fried foods
- Alcohol
- Tobacco smoke
- Pesticides
- Air pollutants
- Metabolic acidosis via excess stress in any form.

Does your <u>Diet</u> and <u>Exercise</u> program reduce the generation of excess ROS?

<u>NOTE:</u>

1. Not all calories are created equally
2. Not all exercise is created equal
3. Not all foods are created equal

Our success is our ability to **differentiate the effects** and **feed the need** of what we do in life.

Is your pattern of exercise, nutrition, stress and lifestyle toxic?

Free radicals- reactive oxygen species ROS are generated via various endogenous systems, as a result of exposure to different physiochemical conditions or pathological states brought on by poor food and lifestyle selection.

Proper metabolic function dictates a need to **balance** of free radicals and antioxidants in our lives. This **<u>BALANCE</u>** is what separates **M360** from other programs and a landscape of misinformation, false promises and chronic disease. We cannot get rid of them, nor would it be healthy to do so, but we must learn to better manage them with the tools of Lifestyle- Physical Activity- Diet & Stress management.

M360 is performed in small groups of like minded individuals willing to **LEARN** how to **CHANGE** their health and wellness landscape and start enjoying:

Metabolic Fitness for LIFE!

If free radical- ROS overwhelms our metabolic ability to down regulate them, oxidative stress (OS) will follow. Loss of metabolic balance and increasing inability to regulate free radical ROS will adversely affect lipids, proteins, DNA triggering a number of chronic diseases.

Oxidative stress is the over production of free radical ROS and our metabolic inability to counteract their detrimental effects with antioxidants sourced, internally (endogenous), and externally (exogenous).

Are <u>YOU</u> overly oxidized and inflamed? _____

How would you know?

- What is your hs-CRP?
- Is it above 1.5?
- Yes or No?

We do not have to stumble around in the dark anymore, so why do we? We can take action and take action **TODAY** to correct Oxidative Stress, and with it Inflammation and Disease. **<u>So why don't we?</u>**

Are we <u>Ignorant,</u> <u>Stupid</u> or just <u>Lazy?</u>

Remember:

- We are ignorant when we do not know better!
- We are stupid if we know better and do it anyway!
- Since you are here reading this- you are intelligent, and motivated to get on the right track to changing your health and life forever. **Congratulations!**

Revelation and Revolution of ROS

As more and more knowledge and understanding of free radicals and reactive oxygen species (ROS) is revealed there tends to be the birth of a revolution that promises a new age of discovery into: Oxidative health and, chronic disease management. **M360** is part of that revolution.

Under certain situations oxygen, which is required for life, can have negative oxidative effects on our body. ROS (Reactive Oxygen Species) are responsible for most of these harmful effects of oxygen. Oxidative stress (OS) and antioxidants have become commonly used terms in modern discussions relating to chronic disease.

We have established that the food we eat and the air we breathe have a lot to do with how well we support both our **endogenous** and **exogenous** ability to reduce excess Oxidation and Inflammation and with it Conditions of Chronic Disease.

Think about that for a minute…

- **The foods we eat and the air we breathe, support what we do, how we do it, and influence our level of wellness, performance and healthspan.**

We have a choice and the more we arm ourselves with simple truth and understanding of how our body works the better off we will be.

It all comes down to **what we choose to do**, or have to do in our next 16 waking hours, how we feed it- and how we recover from it, to do it again. **This is your <u>LIFE</u>!**

Make **<u>NO MISTAKE</u>** about it, **M360** is here to help **<u>YOU</u>** find a better way to reduce **Oxidation** and **Inflammation** and with it improve you **Quality of Life**, by enhancing your performance and reducing or even eliminating the chances of **<u>YOU</u>** having to **<u>SUFFER</u>** through unnecessary **<u>CHRONIC DISEASE!</u>**

Are <u>YOU</u> ready to take that simple step? _____

It appears that under conditions of elevated oxidant load, and moderate exercise- ingestion of antioxidant functional foods and other nutritional supplements may boost our antioxidant reserves- which will assist our body's ability to:

1. Keep oxidative stress responses under control
2. Lower our inflammatory response to life

Does your Diet and Physical Activity Support or Sabotage your ROS defense?

The role of oxidative stress (OS) has been positioned in many conditions including:

- Atherosclerosis
- Cancer
- Respiratory Disease
- Process of aging

Oxidative stress makes a significant contribution to all inflammatory diseases. What are we doing about it? _____

Consistently high levels of Oxidative Stress can lead to the oxidation of lipids and proteins. Oxidation of LDL cholesterol can be deadly!

Free Radical Oxidation, Aging & Dietary Defense

- Our bodies fighting a constant metabolic war to keep from aging. *Are we helping our body or sabotaging its efforts?* _____
- Studies tell us that pathological changes associated with aging are sourced in the free radical damage of our cells. *Does your diet reduce damage?*
- A simple reduction of free radicals or diminished production rate of ROS could reduce and delay the oxidative process of aging. *Does your Diet/Nutrition regime promote or reduce OS?*
- Nutraceutical antioxidants and <u>OUR</u> choice to consume them can retard the aging process and prevent chronic disease.

What <u>Functional Foods</u> defend <u>YOU</u> against OS?

Increased oxidative stress is a metabolic process that occurs during the process of aging. **Antioxidant stimulus** has been shown to significantly down grade the effects of this **oxidative damage** associated with our advancing age. Consider these points in your own journey of choice:

- Free radicals can dramatically increase our rate of aging.
- Free radical damage is preventable via- an adequate defense with antioxidants.
- Antioxidant nutrients can contribute to an enhanced quality of health and life.
- Recent research indicates that antioxidant positively influence life span.

What is an Antioxidant?

Antioxidants are molecules stable enough to provide an electron to a roaming free radical neutralize it, and reduce its ability to inflict metabolic cellular damage.

- Antioxidants are free radical scavengers that protect us free radical cellular damage.
- Antioxidants interact with free radicals to terminate metabolically –detrimental- chain- reactions, before vital molecules get damaged.
- Glutathione, and Ubiquinol, are a few antioxidants, produced endogenously during the normal metabolism of our body.

What's in your Pantry!

There are several enzyme systems that scavenge free radicals, within our body, however principle micronutrient antioxidants are:

- Vitamin E (α-tocopherol),
- Vitamin C (ascorbic acid)
- B-carotene.

These nutrients must be supplied via our diet- as we cannot manufacture these micronutrients alone.

Are <u>YOU</u> supplying the Antioxidants your body <u>NEEDS</u>? _____

Antioxidants act as:

- Radical scavengers
- Hydrogen donors
- Electron donors
- Peroxide decomposers
- Singlet oxygen quenchers
- Enzyme inhibitors
- Synergist
- Metal-chelating agents

Does your Lifestyle support healthy production of endogenous antioxidants?

The more toxic we are, the poorer our nutrition is, the less of these endogenous antioxidants get produced.

- Exogenous sources of antioxidants are also critical, such as
  - ○ Functional Foods, polyphenols, flavonoids...
  - ○ Vitamins C, A, E, D, selenium and many others.

Dynamics of Functional Foods with Nutraceutical Value

"Functional Foods" are defined as food products that have an added positive health benefit.

- Functional foods are necessary for life as a source to assist mental and physical well-being.
- Functional foods contribute to the prevention and reduction of risk factors for chronic diseases while enhancing specific physiological function.

Food can be regarded as "functional" if it is demonstrated to beneficially affect one or more target functions in the body, relative to well being and performance- whilst lowering the risk of a disease.

- Beneficial effects are considered the promotion of our state of well being, health, fitness and a reduction of risk toward the process of disease.

Functional Whole Foods

Functional Whole Foods such as broccoli, carrots, and tomatoes for example, are considered functional foods because of their high contents of metabolically active, health promoting- components:

- **Sulforaphane-** found in cruciferous vegetables such as:
  - ○ Brussels Sprouts, Broccoli, Cabbage, Cauliflower, and Kale
  - ○ Nutraceutical values include:

- antioxidant
- antimicrobial
- anti-inflammatory
- anti-aging
- neuroprotective
- antidiabetic

- **B-carotene-** carotenoids are very potent natural antioxidants! Found in **"Colorful Vegetables & Fruit"**:
  ○ Carrots, Yams, Spinach, Kale, Tomato's
    - Carotenoids
    - Eye Health
    - Cardiovascular Health
    - Skin Health

- **Lycopene-** belongs to a group of pigments known as carotenoids and is considered a phytochemical. This phytochemical occurs naturally in tomatoes and tomato-based products possessing the highest bioavailable concentrations of lycopene. Studies have indicated that Lycopene can upregulate the antioxidant response element (ARE).

- Lycopene has been shown to activate cellular enzymes, like glutathione providing another way of protecting our cells against reactive oxygen species ROS. So eat your tomatoes and spaghetti sauce!

Preparation of Tomatoes: Heated tomatoes are the most bioavailable source of lycopene and are best available to our body when they are sautéed in a meal that provides a small amount of fat. When tomatoes are heated and mixed with olive oil or avocado oil for example, lycopene levels increase substantially vs. unheated tomatoes. I eat tomato with Avocado, Olive Oil, Salt and Pepper and a twist of lemon or lime.

- Other sources of Lycopene are:
  ○ Watermelon, Papaya, Pink Grapefruit, Guava, Red Cabbage, Asparagus, Mango, Red Peppers.

- Defends against Prostate Cancer
- Heart Disease
- Breast Cancer

What is the Nutraceutical value of the Food you EAT?

Nutraceutical is defined: "Functional Whole Foods or parts of foods that provide health benefits, including the prevention and treatment of chronic disease."

There is a huge amount of scientific literature that consistently links consumption of diets rich in vegetables and fruits with reduced risk of the big three killers of man we identified in Section 1:

- Heart Disease -23.4% of total deaths
- Cancer -22.5% of total deaths
- Chronic lower respiratory disease -5.6% of total deaths.

Raw vegetables, green vegetables, allium vegetables, carrots, tomatoes, cruciferous vegetables, and spices are the types of fruits, vegetables, and spices that most often protective us against the **Big 3 Killers** listed above!

Is your diet rich in Functional Foods with Nutraceutical Value? _____

Functional whole foods that aid in the prevention and treatment of disease(s) or disorder(s) are referred to nutraceuticals. Join us in making sure you always have a long list of Functional Whole Foods available in your garden, refrigerator and pantry.

What are Polyphenols?

Naturally occurring Polyphenols compounds are found in fruits, vegetables, cereals and some beverages such as green tea or – coffee.

To simplify our journey through the grocery store it should be noted that 1/3of all polyphenols in our average human diet come from:

1. Coffee
2. Tea
3. Blueberries
4. Cranberries
5. Raspberries
6. Strawberries
7. Pomegranate juice
8. Lettuce
9. Spinach
10. Dark Chocolate

Tea and Coffee

Our morning coffee and tea provide a good portion of our daily intake of antioxidants and is part of a healthy day- so long as you **DO NOT** drown your drink in SUGAR, and HIGH FRUCTOSE CORN SYRUP! If you do add a little sweet stuff, add some heavy cream or MCT oil to counter the insulin reaction. Here are some antioxidant content comparison coffee, tea and cocoa- in terms of available antioxidants:

- Coffee 7-10 grams   150-300 TAC mg/g
- Green Tea 2 grams   150-300 TAC mg/g
- Cocoa 10 grams   200-250 TAC mg/g

All three commons source of antioxidants are rich in Polyphenols.

Flavonoids are the major source of polyphenols in the average diet.

Note: Polyphenols are not all flavonoids however all flavonoids are polyphenols.

What are Flavonoids?

Flavonoids are a group of bioactive compounds that are extensively found in plant based foods. Regular consumption of flavonoids contributes to a reduced risk of a number of neurodegenerative disorders and chronic diseases. Flavonoids act at the molecular level producing antioxidant effects, as well as modulating several key enzymatic pathways.

Regardless of <u>HOW</u> you classify these subjects

Polyphenols and Flavonoids are worth understanding, what they are, and how you can implement them into your diet to improve your **LIFE!** You must employ them to work for your health today!

<u>Is your Diet full of Whole- Functional Foods- Rich in Nutraceutical Value?</u>

The major active nutraceutical ingredients in plants are flavonoids

Flavonoids and Polyphenols are antioxidants, and metal chelators that have been recognized to possess:

- Anti-inflammatory
- Antiallergic
- Hepatoprotective
- Antithrombotic
- Antiviral
- Anticarcinogenic activities.

Here are some of the ingredients that make food functional:

- Dietary fibers
- Vitamins
- Minerals
- Antioxidants
- Oligosaccharides

- Essential fatty acids (omega-3)
- Probiotic bacteria cultures
- Prebiotic foods.

Unlike in west many cultures of medicine around the world believe that complex diseases can be treated with a combination of medicinal plants and natural solutions.

Medicinal Plants and Natural Solutions

Some medicinal plants and dietary constituents having functional attributes are spices such as:

- Onion
- Garlic
- Mustard
- Red chilies
- Turmeric
- Clove
- Cinnamon
- Saffron
- Curry leaf
- Green tea
- Ginger

Are these medicinal plants part of your diet? _____

What would happen to Pharmaceutical Sales in the United States- if **more** people were to eat a complete **Diet of Functional Whole Foods-** rich in **Nutraceuticals** while following a specific regiment of **Feel Good Exercise** as prescribed in Section 2?

_____

Why isn't the power of the US Media asking this question and showing us the numbers- and outlining the solutions as we are here? _____

Your Diet and hs C - reactive protein levels (hs-CRP)

hs C-reactive protein (hs CRP) is an inflammatory marker easily checked by blood test to determine total levels of inflammation in the body. hs CRP is produced by the liver; it becomes elevated with a variety of inflammatory conditions, including digestive, heart and joint problems.

If you have an hs- CRP higher than 1.5 doesn't it make sense to start employing Anti- Oxidant: Exercise, Food and Stress Management into your life TODAY, to lower your silent inflammation?

M360 can lower your CRP and with it a cascade of good events will be free to follow. It is up to you to break out of the corner you have painted yourself into and start enjoying the cascade of wonderful metabolic benefits to enjoy:

Metabolic Fitness for Life

Gut health can determine an individual's overall health.

The human gut has the following functions:

- Breaks food into nutrients
- Stimulate the absorption of nutrients into our blood through intestinal walls
- Defends us from foreign and toxic molecules entering our bloodstream

Gut malfunction can have a direct negative impact on human health.

Probiotics and Gut Health

The use of supplemental, exogenous probiotics has a long association with our state of gut health, overall well-being, and human performance. To understand the role that probiotics may have in influencing health, it is important to have an appreciation of the roles of the normal intestinal micro biome (commensal microbiota). The human gastrointestinal tract is host to over 500 bacterial species, these microbiota form a virtual bioreactor facilitating:

- Digestion
- Nutrient provision
- Shaping of our immune system

Our intestinal bacteria weigh up to 1 kg.

- The ratio of bacterial cells outnumbers human cells is 3:1.
- The bacterial genome may outnumber the human genome by 100:1.

Nutritional factors including several B vitamins, vitamin K, folate, and short chain fatty acids are produced by these bacteria.

How is your Gut Health?

Poor Gut health has a direct negative impact on our metabolic health. **M360** focuses on the role of:

1. Functional Whole Foods
2. Nutraceuticals
3. Food supplements in intestinal health

Human Gut Dynamics, Prebiotics and Probiotics

The Definition of a **prebiotic** is:

- Prebiotics are non-digestible food ingredients that stimulate the growth, or activity of a number of bacteria in our colon, and thus improves our health as a bacterial host

The definition of a **probiotic** is:

- Probiotic is a live microbe supplement that beneficially affects our metabolism as the host while improving our intestinal balance.

Prebiotics and probiotics help regulate our gut microbiota and immune system. Current studies suggest that the composition and function of our gut microbiota- are improved by the supplementation of prebiotics and probiotics.

Metabolic disorders are associated with an increased risk of morbidity and mortality. The underlying point of **M360** is to increase healthspan and reduce morbidity so it is critical to recognize the important role-intestinal microbiota play in the development of Cardio Vascular Disease (CVD) by influencing:

- Body weight,
- Pro-inflammatory activity
- Insulin resistance

The human gut is populated by a wide array of bacterial species, bearing important:

- Metabolic Support
- Immune Functions
- Metabolic effects on our nutritional health status.

Probiotics are **living micro-organisms,** which exert health benefits beyond basic nutrition'. Probiotics are loosely known as live microorganisms belonging to natural biota with low or no pathogenicity (ability to cause harm), but with functions of importance to the health and well being of the host.

Probiotics- are evaluated in four areas of human application in regards to affect on:

1. **Metabolism**
2. **Chronic intestinal inflammatory and functional disorders**
3. **Infections**
4. **Allergy.**

Research has confirmed that the effects of supplemental probiotics on human health are positive, and well defined.

Even more studies suggest that probiotics have beneficial effects on:

- **Fatigue**
- **Osteoporosis**
- **Aging**
- **Obesity**

Prebiotics are a diverse group of carbohydrate ingredients, ONLY -non-digestible oligosaccharides such as **inulin** fulfill the criteria to be classified as a true prebiotic.

Inulin and Oligofructose

These obscure babies belong to a class of carbohydrates known as fructans. Inulin and oligofructose are functional food ingredients that have been known to improve health and reduce our risk of many diseases. They work by stimulating our immune and digestive system of effectively decreasing levels of pathogenic (harmful) bacteria in our intestine. Inulin and Oligofructose have some of the following effects on our life:

- Constipation is relieved with improved motility (+fluid movement)

- Reduced risk of osteoporosis
- Improved mineral absorption —calcium in particular
- Lower serum levels of triglycerides
- Lower fatty acids in the liver, thus reducing the risk of atherosclerosis.

Good health is dependent on healthy gut bifidobacteria in our large intestine and is essential for sustainable diseases prevention.

- The main strategy of **M360** is the **prebiotic** approach – we must supply what our Healthy- Gut Microbiota needs to do its job. We have the opportunity to make better carbohydrate selections and provide the necessary substrates our gut needs for optimal growth of healthy indigenous bifidobacteria.
- Effective carbohydrates (inulin and oligofructose) must reach our colon **undigested** and **unabsorbed.** Once there, they must be utilized by the bacteria population to proliferate.

Examples of Functional Foods with Prebiotic Nutraceutical Inulin value are:

- Chicory Root
- Asparagus
- Garlic
- Onion

Regardless of how you incorporate inulin into your diet, our body uses fiber in the same way. Once it arrives in our gut intact- it acts as a fertilizer for healthy bacteria. Scientific consensus it that inulin will positively affect and balance bacteria in our gut.

Chicory Root is the King of Inulin

Chicory root has a long standing reputation as a cleansing medicinal herb. Ancient Romans used the root to help purify the blood. Ancient Egyptians also consumed the root to clean the blood and detoxify the liver. Medieval monks raised the plants and it is widely used in Europe. Even in southern states like New Orleans (Confederate soldiers drank it during the Civil War, getting in at the ports) it's a coffee substitute.

Health-Boosting Benefits of Chicory

- Chicory root supports digestion, and the breakdown/metabolism of fats by increasing bile production
- It contains **inulin** which is food (a.k.a. prebiotic, a soluble fiber that people cannot digest) for **beneficial digestive flora** (a.k.a. probiotics)—boosting immunity
- Inulin can **regulate blood sugar levels** and **pulls toxins from the body** when we visit the bathroom
- Chicory is full of **antioxidants**
- Chicory will help to **reduce silent inflammation** in the body
- Studies show that it's **antibacterial** and **antifungal**
- Helps **reduce heart rate** and has been used use in the treatment of tachycardia (rapid heartbeat), arrhythmia and fibrillation
- Helps **boost digestion** and relieve constipation
- I have personally seen it help lower the Heart Rate Cost's of Specific Power (wattage workload) on my smart trainer. Much like Beet Juice and Dark Chocolate. Vasodilators that reduce the Oxygen Cost's of Physical Workload.

These fructans modulate the hormonal level of insulin and glucagon, thereby:

- Regulating carbohydrate and lipid metabolism by lowering the blood glucose levels; they are also effective in
- Lowering the blood urea and uric acid levels (any Gout Sufferers out there?

Simple Application:

I use a loose tea screen that contains my roasted Chicory, about a tablespoon, and submerge it into my morning coffee. I find it adds substance to my coffee in terms of flavor and of course gives me a great shot of inulin along with all the benefits we have discussed.

Probiotics and prebiotics share unique roles the manipulation of populations our human GUT microbiota that colonize our GI tract. Consumption of probiotics along with prebiotics has health benefits that include:

- Enhanced **immune function**
- Improved **colonic integrity**
- Decreased **intestinal infections** both incidence and duration
- Down-regulated **allergic** response
- Improved **digestion** and **elimination** -**transit time**

Imbalance of Intestinal Microbial Flora in Today's World

Modern lifestyles impose stress on our metabolic systems genetically adapted over millions of years. Our consumption of food containing microorganisms has dramatically reduced, causing a lack of metabolic immune education.

- This lack of **immune education** retards and impairs our **immune system** resulting in inflammatory damage, allergy and/or autoimmunity.

Background Summary INFO on Probiotics

Probiotics: what the studies show

1. Hundreds of trillions of bacteria live in our large intestine
2. Most of our bacteria are beneficial, and perform vital metabolic functions

3. Our bacterial buddies keep BAD bacteria at bay, whilst helping us with optimal immunity, better digestion, and better nutrient absorption- even protecting us with anticancer effects.

You may ask yourself as I do: *"Does taking probiotics in foods or capsules make a difference to our health—even if we are already healthy? The answer appears to be a resounding* **YES***!*

Here's a look at the evidence

Studies over the last 50 years have clearly shown that diets dominated by, vegetables, some fruits and dietary fibers (plant based foods) **prevent** and **reduce** the risk of **chronic diseases** (e.g. cardiovascular diseases, obesity, diabetes) and promote human health and performance.

The generation of scientific research linking foods of plant origin and health worldwide has resulted in acknowledgement that:

Plant Based Diets have anti-oxidant and other healthy properties such as:

- **Inulin**
- **Nitrates**
- **Polyphenols**
- **Flavonoids**
- **Phytonutrients**

Are you beginning to piece it all together how our **GUT** Flora is the base of our Immune System and how the health of our **GUT** can positively or negatively affect our ability to digest and metabolize food for energy?

Do the foods you eat provide the Prebiotics and Probiotics you need?

Are you beginning to see that the ability of our **GUT**, to optimize its function can be dictated by us **PROVIDING** the nutraceutical contents of plants- available to grow the flora we need- to make the food we eat, and the air we breathe- bio available for our metabolism to utilize and thrive?

Robust Health is strongly linked to a Plant Based Diet

High dietary intake of vegetables, spices, herbs, fruits, wild caught fish and grass fed beef is strongly associated with reduced risk of developing chronic diseases, such as cancer and cardiovascular diseases (CVD), which as you know- are the highest causes of death in United States and in most industrialized countries.

One Third of All Cancer Deaths can be avoided with <u>ONE</u> Intervention!

Research supports that- one-third of all cancer deaths in industrialized countries could be avoided through appropriate dietary formulations. This statement suggests that dietary behavioral changes, such as increasing consumption of vegetables, fruits, spices, herbs and related changes in lifestyle are practical strategies for significant reduction of the incidence of cancer as well as a whole list of chronic conditions that lead to chronic disease.

Are you <u>READY</u> to check your list's and make some changes?

There is a huge amount of scientific literature- consistently linking consumption of diets rich in vegetables, spices, herbs and fruits with reduced risk of:

- **Heart disease**
- **Respiratory disease**
- **Cancer**

Based on numerous human studies- similar effects of **Plant Based Diets** are consistent for cancers of the stomach, esophagus, lung, oral cavity, pancreas, and colon. **RAW VEGETABLES** appear to be the most protective against cancer such as:

- **Allium Vegetables**
  a. Onion
  b. Garlic
  c. Asparagus
- **Root Vegetables**
  a. Chicory
  b. Beets
  c. Turmeric
  d. Ginger
- **Green vegetables**
  a. Kale
  b. Romaine Lettuce
  c. Dandelion Greens
- **Cruciferous vegetables**
  a. Brussels Sprouts
  b. Broccoli
  c. Cabbage
- **Herbs and Spices** have been identified as sources of various phytochemicals, which possess powerful antioxidant activity thus, herbs and spices have an important role in antioxidant/anti-inflammatory defense. Herbs and spices and composite herbal medicines are among the categories that contain the most antioxidants.
  a. Ginger
  b. Turmeric
  c. Cinnamon
  d. Chili
  e. Green Tea (Not really herbal, but very antioxidant)

Diet -Blood Pressure and Athletic Performance

- Optimal blood pressure is critical to our prevention of heart disease, stroke and kidney disease.
- Blood pressure is influenced by many factors:
  - Atherosclerosis
  - Imbalances in our hormone system that regulates blood pressure and fluid balance
  - Hyper-insulinemia (excess levels of insulin circulating in the blood)

Consequently, a general nutritional plan to minimize hypertension risk includes attaining and maintaining a healthy body weight; consuming a diet rich in calcium, phosphorus, and magnesium; and nitrates.

- Dietary nitrate has been demonstrated to have a range of beneficial vascular effects:
  - Reducing blood pressure,
  - Inhibiting platelet aggregation,
  - Preserving or improving endothelial dysfunction,
  - Enhancing exercise performance in healthy individuals and patients with peripheral arterial disease.
- Nitric oxide (NO), is a potent vasodilator critical in maintaining vascular homeostasis, and has been proven to reduce blood pressure.
- Dietary nitrate consumption is also associated with improvements in vascular function.
- 85% of dietary nitrate is derived from vegetables

Common Key Sources of Dietary Nitrate are:

- Arugula Greens
- Spinach
- Raw Beets

Question to the Healthcare World?

When a patient population is sick with conditions of chronic disease to the point of $2.9 Trillion out of a Total $3.2 Trillion in total health care, **WHY** is there **NOT** a Program and Place for these Patient Populations to go and learn the value of foods and **HOW** they can prevent, and even reverse conditions such as **High Blood Pressure** for example- with **NATURAL WHOLE FOODS?**

M360 is on a **MISSION** to penetrate this ignorance and stupidity with small personalized clinics to address small groups of 5-6 people with 8-12- week, 15- modality- Total Immersion Blocks of Learning, Exercising, and Nutrition Planning and Stress management techniques for everyday life. We **CAN** and **MUST** change our approach.

Dietary Nitrates and Platelet function

Platelets influence vascular disease through their interaction with the vessel wall, and play a significant part in the development of coronary syndromes. Nitric oxide from dietary nitrates has been shown to inhibit platelet adhesion to the endothelium (Blood Vessel Walls) and platelet aggregation (cluster).

Blood Pressure and Dietary Nitrate

Dietary nitrate (found in green leafy vegetables and in beetroot) is now recognized to be an important source of nitric oxide (NO), via the nitrate-nitrite-NO pathway. Dietary nitrate confers several cardiovascular beneficial effects on blood pressure, platelets, endothelial function, mitochondrial efficiency and exercise. While this pathway may now seem obvious, its realization followed a rather tortuous course over two decades.

Research published in 2014 showed that a diet including inorganic nitrates from **red beets** and green leafy vegetables can **lower blood pressure**; improve the ability to, and the duration of, exercise; boost oxygen delivery to the heart; and enhance general health.

Exercise/Athletic performance

A fundamental principle of exercise physiology is that during exercise, the oxygen cost, is predictable for a given submaximal work rate. A simple **M360** training session example is **Power Production (wattage)** on a Bike vs. % MHR (Max Heart Rate) cost expressed in terms of **Percentage (%) of Max Heart Rate** to produce a given power (intensity) output for a given period of time (duration).

- **Sample: 200 watts @ 80% of MHR for 20 minutes.**

Studies tested the effects of 3-days of dietary nitrate supplementation with beetroot juice as a source of **Nitric Oxide** (NO), on exercise performance they surprisingly found that:

- Nitric Oxide consumption resulted the substantial reduction of oxygen cost's during submaximal exercise (between 45–80% of Max Heart Rate) with no effect on plasma lactate concentration.
- These Studies suggest that exercise becomes more efficient and the oxygen cost is reduced for same workload prior to consumption of Nitric Oxide.
- In practical **M360** terms this research suggests that beetroot juice, rich in Nitric Oxide- has been shown to reduce the oxygen cost of same work load.

This would be simplified as follows:

<u>Pre</u> Beetroot Juice:

- **Sample: 200 watts @ 75% of MHR for 20 minutes**

<u>Post</u> Beetroot Juice:

- **Sample: 200 watts @ 70% of MHR for 20 minutes.**

Same athlete, same bike, and same wattage – BETTER PERFORMANCE!

You be the judge on the power of dietary nitrate found in Red Beet Juice, which tastes great by the way. I also have personal experience with these benefits and performance enhancement to my own competitions, also from Chicory Root and Dark Chocolate!

Studies show that Nitrate supplementation also reduced maximal oxygen consumption found similar results with beetroot juice which reduced the increase in pulmonary oxygen uptake during moderate exercise by ~19%, reduced the slow component of O_2 uptake during severe exercise, and increased time to exhaustion.

- 20% reduction in oxygen cost due to beetroot juice ingestion was due to a reduction in ATP (Adenosine Triphosphate) cost of muscle force at both low and high intensity exercise.
- There was also a 16% improvement in the time to task failure during severe exercise.
- The duration of these beneficial effects of **beetroot juice** on exercise performance and blood pressure lowering range from-
  ◦ Acute effects at 2.5 h
  ◦ Sustained effects over 15 days.

Do you drink Beet Juice? _____

Using a nitrate-depleted beetroot juice as placebo, it was demonstrated that:

- It was the nitrate content of the active juice, rather than other components such as betaine or polyphenols that was responsible for the improvements in the reduced O_2 cost of walking and moderate to severe intensity running and a **15% increase in time-to-exhaustion.**

Other studies have demonstrated acute improvements in power output with nitrate during cycling time trials. Ingestion of **750 ml of beetroot juice over the preceding 24 h** (9.3 mmol nitrate) resulted in reduced muscle and metabolic disruption along with a remarkably restored exercise tolerance and oxidative capacity.

Do you see the Nutraceutical Value of Nitric Oxide in Red Beets?

What are the Nutraceutical Values of the <u>FOOD</u> we <u>EAT</u>?:

- Nutraceuticals aid in the prevention and treatment of disease or other chronic disorders.
- Nutraceuticals assist our body to sustain optimal metabolic function.
- Are we nutraceutically challenged? **ARE YOU!**

Polyunsaturated Fat and Gut Microbiota

Polyunsaturated fatty acids (PUFAs) (which include the omega-3 and omega-6 fatty acids) and phytochemicals also play an important role as healthy dietary bioactive compounds. Phytochemicals (bioactive non-nutrient plant compounds), are being popularized in human nutrition because of their potential effects as:

- **Antioxidants**
- **Anti-inflammatory**
- **Anti-carcinogenic**

Gut microbiota transform and affect the bioavailability and effects of polyphenols. Phytochemicals and their metabolic products may also inhibit pathogenic bacteria while stimulating the growth of beneficial bacteria.

M360 will help you connect Components of Health into your Lifestyle

Interactions between functional food components, such as prebiotics, probiotics, phytochemicals, and intestinal microbiota, have consequences on human health.

Nutraceutical - Functional Food is the Future of <u>REAL</u> Home Healthcare

Real home healthcare is more than some inflamed -overweight person sitting in your living room-laptop computer open and billing insurance companies under the guise of home healthcare. I have personally seen this with my 87 yrs old mother.

Real Home Healthcare will be a qualified- lean- healthy person, who will help stock the home living situation with functional whole foods containing specific nutraceutical values- along with necessary supplements(broadly including probiotics, prebiotics, phytochemicals *etc.*). Homecare will **TARGET** the consumption of appropriate anti-inflammatory diets and healthy eating models, along with simple activities to address specific health issue of the individual client.

Appropriate diet is the precursor to a healthy, properly functioning **Energy Metabolism**. A high performance diet, rich in functional whole food results in the achievement of optimal human physiology, via healthy living; if we do not make these interventions we can expect a cascade of conditions leading to chronic disease.

Get your Greens and Beets: more on the Nutraceutical of Dietary Nitrate

Dietary nitrate has been demonstrated to have a range of beneficial vascular effects, including reducing blood pressure, inhibiting platelet aggregation, preserving or improving endothelial dysfunction, enhancing exercise performance in healthy individuals and patients with peripheral arterial disease.

Plant based diets are associated with lower blood pressure and are associated with a reduced incidence of non-fatal myocardial infarction or fatal coronary heart disease and stroke.

The top plant based dietary sources of nitrate are:

- Red Beets
- Spinach
- Lettuce
- Radish
- Cabbage
- Green Beans
- Cucumber
- Carrots
- Garlic
- Green Peppers

Vascular Effects of Plant Based Dietary Nitrate

Dietary nitrate converted to Nitric Oxide (NO) has been demonstrated to have a range of beneficial vascular effects, including:

- Reducing blood pressure
- Enhancing exercise performance
- Inhibiting platelet aggregation

Nitric oxide (**NO**) is a very strong chemical that causes our blood vessels to relax, which improves blood flow to our organs, muscles, and — most importantly — our heart. Without this **NO**, our capacity to exercise will be reduced leaving us with symptoms of a stiff heart, often expressed as shortness of breath and fatigue.

Caution with all Good Things

Dose is always a factor. There is such a thing as:

"Even Too Much of a Good Thing can be bad"

I once knew gal I ran with at Arizona who drank so much carrot juice she had an orange hue. Probably a little much, don't you think?

Always use your head when discovering the values of functional foods and do your best to get the value of these foods in their most natural presentation.

Example: Apples eat a whole organic well washed apple, complete with a balance of fiber to sugar ratio and not a gallon of apple juice. Let common sense prevail. Same is true for Beets, Carrots as well as other wonderful foods.

The Magic Nutraceuticals of Dark Chocolate, Human Performance & Health

Dark chocolate (DC) is abundant in flavanols which have been reported to increase the bioavailability and bioactivity of nitric oxide (NO). Increasing NO bioavailability is associated with performance enhancing- reduced oxygen cost during submaximal exercise.

Dark Chocolate Research Testing

Smart Trainer cycling tests were performed at 80 % of each clients established Gas Exchange Threshold (GET) for 20-min followed- by a two-minute time-trial (TT), two weeks apart, with **40 g of DC** being consumed daily.

Consistent supplementation of Dark Chocolate (DC) resulted in a higher (GET) Gas Exchange Threshold and improved Time Trial (TT) performance.

Oxygen cost of moderate intensity exercise was reduced with the Ingestion of DC! In other words the **POWER** (wattage output) oxygen and heart rate cost of a given POWER output as measured in Wattage was reduced. Oxygen cost to perform activity-at same intensity- went DOWN!

Dark chocolate (DC), rich in cocoa polyphenols, is shown to have a positive effect on plasma metabolites, hormones, and markers of oxidative stress after prolonged exhaustive exercise. Studies suggest that regular DC intake, up to 40g a day, are associated with:

- Reduced oxidative-stress markers
- Increased mobilization of free fatty acids (FFA)

Cholesterol Tails and Truths?

Get educated on Cholesterol; it is one of the most important substances inside of your body. Put into perspective what is considered **'HIGH'** by conventional standards isn't necessarily high at all, you be the judge? Points to consider:

- Cholesterol is made by your body to protect you, not to kill you. The human body has not evolved to kill itself.
- Your body is constantly trying to do the best that it can given the circumstances. *This is called homeostasis* or *homeostatic control*; the body in a constant attempt to achieve a state of equilibrium, on every level. Are you **SUPPORTING** or **SABOTAGING** your body in this attempt?
- Any competent healthcare provider should evaluate **ALL** of the underlying metabolic situations occurring in our body. What are the **REAL** markers of our Health and Performance we should be addressing?
- We deserve the highest quality healthcare and our providers should work for us diligently! If they aren't seeking metabolic health and wellness via interventions of lifestyle-Exercise-Diet-Stress mgmt. then we should fire them and seek a metabolic collaboration elsewhere.

Cholesterol is not our enemy, it is our friend. Here's what it does:

- Cholesterol gives integrity to every structure of every cell of our body. Low cholesterol levels are often associated with a metabolic- ***catabolic state***, A state where cells are weaker with increased susceptibility to free radical harm.

- **EVERY** steroid hormone, including your adrenal and sex hormones are built from the building blocks of cholesterol.
- In my opinion there is no such thing as a **'bad cholesterol'.** When you consider that every steroid hormone is made of the LDL particles circulating in your blood you would have to agree. Our body is **INCAPABLE** of making steroid hormones without LDL. That's a big one! LDL cholesterol is a fundamental precursor in our body's ability to repair damaged cells and make new ones.
- The assimilation of fat soluble Vitamins: A, D, E and K would not happen without Cholesterol. Bile and bile acids join forces with cholesterol in the assimilation of these powerful fat soluble nutrients.
- Cholesterol acts as a potent free radical scavenging- antioxidant and protects our cells from oxidative damage.
- Cholesterol repairs damaged cells as a metabolic nutrient.

Some Evidence Suggests High LDL in Fat Adapted Athletes. In the absence of stored body **fat** the body produces more **LDL** to satisfy the need for energy. ... **Elevated** blood **cholesterol** in a **fat-adapted** athlete signifies an up-regulated **metabolism** that is geared to meet **higher** energy demands associated with diet, activity and endurance.

Total Cholesterol (common view) Question this!

What's your cholesterol level? Mine is **262** mg/dl

- Desirable: Lower than 240 mg/dl
- Borderline high: 200-239 mg/dl
- High-risk: Higher than 240 mg/dl

HDL Cholesterol

Reduced risk for heart disease is associated with higher HDL levels. HDL-C is known as the "good" cholesterol and is believed to remove excess cholesterol from coronary arteries.

What's your HDL cholesterol level? Mine is **89** mg/dl

- Desirable: Higher than 35 mg/dl

Triglyceride

Triglyceride helps us to store fat in the body. Elevated levels of triglyceride may play a role in the increased risk of heart disease.

What's your triglyceride level? Mine is **53** mg/dl yours_____

- Desirable: Lower than 250 mg/dl

Risk Factors for Heart Disease

Cholesterol level is just one view of risk factors for CVD. There is another way to assess your risk for CVD, based on our inflammation, and oxidation potential.

The main factors we will target with **M360** as risk factors and of cardiovascular disease, as well as other health conditions are:

- Cardio hs-CRP (mine is **.43** mg/L)
- Insulin Resistance (mine is **<25** on LP-IR Score)
- Triglycerides (mine is **53** mg/dL)
- HDL-C (mine is **87** mg/dL)
- **Should I recognize CRP, Insulin Resistance, Triglycerides and HDL-C as the Markers of <u>MY HEALTH</u> and lifestyle components to modify or <u>Total Cholesterol</u>?**
- **Should I go on a Statin Drug for the rest of my life, or educate myself on proper- moderate, reference point physical activity- along with consumption of nitrate rich,**

nutrient rich, functional, antioxidant -whole foods- high in nutraceutical, value along with proper sleep and recovery?

Elevated hs-CRP is a major indicator of CVD risk when elevated. Also called Cardiovascular C - reactive protein you want this test to come back 1.5 or less.

Elevated Triglycerides and low HDL-c are other indicators of cardiovascular disease risk factor, especially if correlated with High Cardio CRP and Insulin Resistance.

One of the primary ways that elevated insulin can increase a person's CVD risk is through **insulin resistance**. When the cells become over-exposed to this crucial hormone, insulin resistance takes place. Insulin resistance will also cause a high excretion of magnesium as well as retention of sodium. Both of these processes significantly increase one's risk for cardiovascular disease CVD.

Magnesium is a critical electrolyte for vasodilatation and for increasing nitric oxide in the arteries, both of which antagonize cardiovascular disease risk factors.

Diets high in sugar and foods that break down into sugars wreak havoc!

High Glycemic loads will cause a lot of insulin to be released by the pancreas. This is especially true for people, who are very sensitive to sugars and carbohydrates.

If you are at a high risk for CVD, request that these factors be run in your next blood test. If your doctor asks why you are requesting insulin, tell he or she that you are interested in protecting your health rather than taking drugs. If your doctor won't run these tests, then fire your doctor and find someone else who will.

Higher Fat - Lower Carb Diets and Fat Adapted Biomarker Improvement

Low-carbohydrate-high-fat (LCHF) diets have been used as a means of weight loss and control of conditions of chronic disease in several clinical settings. Research suggests that LCHF diets induce metabolic change that can enhance endurance performance.

Fat Adapted Metabolism (Are YOU Fat Adapted?)

Fat Adapted Athletes can achieve the maximal fat oxidation rate of approximately 1.5 g/min with a lower carbohydrate utilization rate and similar muscle glycogen content. This is a metabolic nirvana that optimizes body fat as the prime source of fuel while conserving glycogen for when it is most needed at higher intensity outputs.

Elevated Fat Oxidation

Elevated fat oxidation and glycogen sparing effect of becoming fat adapted can improve endurance and ultra endurance capacities. Fat Adapted metabolic changes can also prevent low performance in late stages of anaerobic interval training-where the anaerobic metabolism becomes most important.

Fat Adapted Macro Nutrient Overview

Fat Adapted diets, referred to as ketogenic diets; usually contain less than 20% of energy from Net-carbohydrate, 50%-70% of energy coming from fat, with variable amounts of quality protein. I usually range between 50-70% Good Fat and 10-20% lower glycemic load –fibrous carbohydrate leaving the balance in quality protein.

Studies show that consuming a Fat Adapted diet over months and years does NOT lead to any metabolic imbalances provided there is sufficient total energy and adequate amounts of protein. Contrary to ideas that a high fat diet would increase the risk for obesity, and cardiovascular disease, Fat Adapted diets have been shown to actually reduce these metabolic risk factors.

Fat Mass and Lean Mass in Fat Adapted diets

Studies with overweight women have proven that Fat Adapted diets in combination with moderate resistance training could reduce fat mass (FM) while maintaining lean body mass (LM).

Resistance training in combination with higher-carbohydrate diets increased Lean Mass, however did NOT reduce Fat Mass. Fat Adapted diets, along with moderate resistance training, will maintain lean mass and reap the benefits of loss in fat mass as well as overall body weight. The key is to reduced insulin response; improve Strength to Weight Ratio, to support efficient mitochondrial ATP production or **"Energy"**!

Fat Oxidation and Intensity of Activity

It is a well-known fact that maximal fat oxidation is reached at moderate-intensity exercise corresponding to:

- 59-64% VO_{2max} (**75-80%** mhr) in endurance-trained individuals, and
- 47-52% VO_{2max} (**65-70%** mhr) in the general population.

Any CPET test will clearly show under normal conditions that fat oxidation rate drops dramatically above this inflection point of exercise intensity.

Athletic Performance with a Fat Adapted Metabolism

Fat Adapted Diets resulted in **higher fat oxidation rates** and a **lower carbohydrate utilization rate.** The result is simple: Utilize Fat for fuel and conserve Glycogen for times of emergency when it is needed most in the case of fight or flight.

Fat Adapted Benefits

FAT ADAPTED diets produce many metabolic benefits; however these 2 are the key:

- **Higher rates of fat oxidation**
- **Lower rates of glycogenolysis and carbohydrate oxidation.**

Studies prove that Fat Adapted endurance athletes reach the maximal fat oxidation rate of approximately 1.5 g/min at **80-85% mhr** (ATP Training Transition point to LBP) for our **M360** comparison. At **M360** we fine tune the **FEEL GOOD** transition point of exercise- between **Nothing** and **TOO MUCH!**

The bottom line is we can get more energy from our biggest -**source of energy**- which is **FAT**. We unlock our savings account.

Efficient FAT Energy to FUND our ACTIVITES

Ultra-endurance athletes who consumed fat adapted diets 70% fat with 20% energy from carb for at least 6-months achieved higher peak exercise workloads than high carb athletes on HCLF diet.

Fat-adapted athletes also showed a higher fat oxidation rate and a lower carbohydrate consumption during prolonged exercise <80% MHR.

Plant based Diet to reduce and prevent Atherogenesis (Atherogens)

A plant-based diet is increasingly becoming recognized as a healthier alternative to a diet laden with meat. Polyphenols derived from dietary plant intake have protective effects on vascular endothelial cells, possibly as antioxidants that prevent the oxidation of low-density lipoprotein.

Recent literature suggests that lifestyle management that includes a diet of mostly plants may help prevent and reverse Coronary Artery Disease (CAD). Plant-based nutrition is the predominant consumption of plant-based, whole foods to obtain macronutrients (carbohydrates, protein, and fats), micronutrients (vitamins and minerals), and bioactive components (eg, flavonoids, plant sterols, polyphenols) that optimize body function. It is a conscious and mindful decision to maximize the health benefits per calorie while minimizing potential harmful exposures.

Vascular Endothelial Cell (VEC) Injury

VECs play a key role in the regulation of vascular homeostasis, and increasing evidence suggests that alterations in endothelial function contribute to the development of disease (pathogenesis) and clinical expression of Coronary Artery Disease (CAD). Causes of initial VEC injury include elevated blood sugar levels, insulin resistance, CRP levels, diabetes, and high blood pressure.

Recent studies- and the THESIS of **M360,** is to show that lifestyle management with physical activity and nutrition, may prevent diabetes; lower blood pressure levels- lower Triglyceride levels, lower CRP, raise HDL and prevent CAD events and death. Therefore, changing to a plant-based diet may decrease CAD mortality by interrupting or reversing the process of atherogenesis (scarring of the arterial wall).

A plant-based diet decreases the risks associated with CAD and may down-regulate inflammation leading to atherogenesis by decreasing the intake of substances found in processed foods, added sugars, oils, and processed meats that promote atherogenesis with a reciprocal increased intake of bioactive substances found in plants that protect the endothelium and inhibit atherogenesis. **Serve and protect or destroy?**

Polyphenols and the Scarring of Blood Vessel Walls

On the basis of cell culture studies, polyphenols may positively affect critical steps and reduce atherogenesis (Scarring of Blood Vessel Walls), including:

- ***LDL oxidation***,
- Nitric oxide release
- Inflammation
- Oxidative stress
- Cell adhesion
- Foam cell formation
- Proliferation of smooth muscle cells
- Platelet aggregation

Flavonoids Join in to protect us from CAD, Vascular tone and Inflammation

- Evidence suggests that individuals with the highest polyphenols intake have modestly reduced risks for CAD.
- There is increasing evidence that flavonoids may have beneficial effects on Vascular Endothelial Cells expressing control of thrombosis, inflammation, and vascular tone.

How is your Vascular Tone? _____

The vascular tone of blood vessels and arteries determine how hard the heart has to work to pump blood throughout the body. When there is no resistance from blood vessels, the heart is able to pump smoothly, reducing the risk of heart disease. The higher the resistance from blood vessels, the harder the heart has to pump, the higher the risk of heart disease. **How hard is your Heart Working?** _____

Polyphenols have beneficial effects that limit platelet adhesion and aggregation that can precipitate acute coronary syndromes after plaque rupture. Overall diet will also influence the effects of risk factors on VEC function.

Studies have shown that vascular endothelial dysfunction is associated with an increased risk of Coronary Artery Disease events. Many interventions known to reduce CAD risk have the ability to reverse endothelial dysfunction.

Proper Exercise and Nutrition Supports Optimal Vascular Tone

Moderate Intensity Exercise of longer Durations- involving the largest Muscle Mass as in activities like:

- Swimming
- Running
- Cycling
- Paddling
- Walking
- Full Body Functional Resistance Training and Yoga

M360 exercise training improves endothelial function by up regulating Nitric Oxide improving protein expression and increasing phosphorylation of enzymes. In simple terms blood flows easier in and out of the heart as well as in and out of all tissue of the body to support increased **Power- Vitality** and **Function.**

Arteries in health and disease

The endothelium is the innermost of the artery's three layers. It produces nitric oxide, which helps keep the artery open and healthy. Plaques have the opposite effect.

Endothelial cells have a crucial role in vascular health, and exercise has an important effect on endothelial cells, endothelial cells also produce *nitric oxide.*

Nitric oxide has two crucial functions.

- It keeps the arterial lining smooth and slippery, preventing white blood cells and platelets from latching on and causing damaging inflammation and artery-blocking blood clots.

- In addition, it **relaxes** the **smooth muscle cells** of the artery wall's middle layer, preventing spasms and keeping arteries open.

Findings suggest that vascular endothelial function can be optimized with lifestyle interventions which can prevent and treat coronary artery disease. **M360** is a simple program that targets and addresses risk factors focusing efforts at every level of life- to optimize all the functions of our body- and help our metabolism out, pretty simple!

Are You Ready to have some Blood Tests? _____

M360 Blood Test Bio Markers for Total Health and Performance:

1. hs -CRP:
2. HDL-C:
3. Triglycerides:
4. Insulin Resistance:

Remember the Top 3- Chronic Diseases that are killing us?

- **One of the best ways to live a longer and better life is to reduce your likelihood of dying from heart disease.**

If we could eliminate heart disease tomorrow, the average life expectancy of every American would increase by an estimated ten years. Although mortality from heart disease has decreased due to medical advances, the incidence of heart disease is on the rise.

Is your Lifestyle Program addressing the Underlying Causes of Heart Disease?

More of us are getting heart disease because we aren't doing enough to address the underlying cause of Heart Disease:

- **Inflammation in the arteries**

Like all silent inflammation, arterial inflammation stems from increased production of "bad" eicosanoids. Rather than pinning your hopes on some new surgery or drug that may, or may not be developed in the future, why not just avoid getting heart disease in the first place?

What Stimulates the Production of "bad" Eicosanoids?

There is a large nutritional myth that we have to consume high amounts of carbohydrates to remain healthy. Research now suggests just the opposite.

- Not only is most of our obesity related to carbohydrate excess, but many of the diseases that plague or society, such as arthritis, cancer, and cardiovascular disease are related to this unhealthy, over carb fed practice.
- Not only should we reduce our carbohydrate intake but we should also carefully select the type of carbohydrates we do eat.

We often times hear the question:

"Are all carbohydrates equal in terms of absorption from the gut?"

To answer is <u>NO</u>!

Carbohydrates are absorbed at highly variable rates.

- Some are absorbed very rapidly, and others slowly. So why does this matter?
  - The rate of absorption of carbohydrates determines the amount of insulin secreted in response from the pancreas.
  - Carbohydrates rapidly absorbed by the gut flood the bloodstream with glucose (all carbohydrates are converted to glucose).

- To handle this immediate load of sugar the pancreas has to secrete a large amount of insulin. Too much- too often and you can become insulin resistant.

Over sixty million Americans generate excess insulin that, in turn, drives blood sugar to levels that can impair brain function. We experience this through intense hunger, anxiety, and tremulousness.

"Will changing our diet early in life prevent neurodegenerative diseases?"

Asking this question makes it very important to note that- food should be viewed as an extremely powerful drug.

Food has the <u>POWER</u> to <u>CHANGE</u> your <u>LIFE</u>!

Is Silent Inflammation Killing your Heart?

- A heart attack is simply the death of the muscle cells in the heart due to a lack of oxygen, caused by a constriction in blood flow.
- If this lack of oxygen is prolonged, enough heart muscle cells die, and your heart attack becomes a fatal one.

There are several things that can cause the stoppage of oxygen flow to the heart.

- A rupture could occur in a piece of unstable plaque lining the artery wall. This causes the activation of platelets, which clump together and block blood flow.
- You could have a spasm in the artery that blocks blood flow to the heart. This may be due to an electrical flutter, which disrupts the synchronized beating and causes the heart to stop functioning altogether.

None of these heart attack causes has much to do with increased cholesterol levels, but they have everything to do with **Silent Inflammation**.

You may be asking yourself, "How can inflammation be silent"?

- Silent inflammation is simply inflammation that falls below the threshold of perceived pain. That's what makes it so dangerous.
- You don't take any steps to stop it as it smolders for years, if not decades, eventually erupting into what we call chronic disease.

A variety of factors forge the linkage between silent inflammation and fatal heart attacks.

1. First of all, pro-inflammatory *eicosanoids inside an unstable plaque can trigger the inflammation that increases the likelihood of rupture.
   a. ***NOTE**: Eicosanoids are simply compounds involved in cellular activity they can be pro-inflammatory or anti-inflammatory.
2. Often these unstable plaques are so small that they can't be detected by conventional technology like an angiogram.
3. When such a plaque bursts, cellular debris is released and platelets rush to the site in an attempt to repair the rupture, just as it would a wound.
4. New blood clots formed from aggregated platelets may plug up the artery, stopping blood flow completely.

This helps explain why many people do not die of heart attacks even though they have highly clogged arteries, whereas others do, even though they have seemingly normal arteries. It all depends on the levels of inflammation in these small, unstable plaques.

Pro-inflammatory eicosanoids act as powerful constrictors of your arteries and can lead to a vasospasm, a potentially fatal cramp or **"charley horse"** that prevents blood flow to the heart.

Lack of sufficient levels of long-chain omega-3 fatty acids (found in fish oil) in the heart muscle can also lead to a fatal heart attack caused by chaotic electric rhythms in the heart. This condition, called sudden death, accounts for more than <u>50 percent</u> of all fatal heart attacks.

Fish Oil and Silent Inflammation

Ultra Refined high-dose fish oil, especially when coupled with improved insulin control, can have a significant role in the prevention and treatment of heart disease.

- By controlling your level of silent inflammation, you can reduce your risk of dying of heart disease to being as rare as it was at the beginning of the twentieth century.

More on Oxidative Stress (OS)

Research studies define oxidative stress (OS) as:

An imbalance of more oxidants than antioxidants

OS is linked with the disruption of metabolic signaling pathways, damage of macromolecules, and the disruption of metabolic homeostasis.

Oxidative stress is directly linked to a balance between the pool of our oxidant and antioxidant mechanisms.

Endogenous and Dietary Antioxidants that support Exercise and Life Activities

Antioxidants can be divided into categories according to specific characteristics.

- **Enzymatic** such as:
  - o Superoxide dismutase (SOD)
  - o Catalase
  - o Glutathione reductase
  - o Glutathione peroxidase (GPX)
- **Non-enzymatic** metabolites such as:
  - o Glutathione
  - o Uric acid
  - o Vitamins
  - o Polyphenols

Regarding their origin, various antioxidants such as glutathione, uric acid, catalase and SOD they are produced endogenously (within our body), whereas others, namely, polyphenols and β-carotene, are obtained from food exogenously (outside of body).

Antioxidants can be divided into:

- **Water-soluble** antioxidants -glutathione, and polyphenols
- **Lipid-soluble** antioxidants -vitamins A and E and lipoic acid.

Anti-Oxidant components that Protect our Health

Oxidative agents and antioxidant mechanisms are in a potential balance. The disturbance of the equilibrium between <u>oxidative mechanisms</u> and <u>antioxidants</u>, in favor of <u>oxidative mechanisms</u>- is referred to as <u>oxidative stress</u>

- *   **Glutathione** is considered one of the most important and powerful **endogenous** antioxidant metabolites and is the first line of defense against reactive oxygen species ROS.

   *   **Polyphenols** on the other hand are considered some of
       the most important and powerful **exogenous** antioxidant
       dietary defense against reactive oxygen species ROS.

Many studies have confirmed beneficial effects of polyphenolic
compounds on our health. It has been demonstrated that consumption
of **polyphenols** results in the prevention of cardiovascular diseases as
well as many conditions of chronic disease.

Do you or have you ever had any Digestive, Heart or Joint Problems?

Research has shown that lowering the levels of inflammation in the body
can greatly reduce the risk of heart attack, stroke, digestive problems
and joint issues.

Inflammation can be reduced with a variety of lifestyle strategies,
including:

   *   Targeting Nutraceutical components of Functional Whole
       Foods.
   *   Improved Heart Rate Variability (HRV)
   *   Improved Fitness as a measure of Strength to Weight Ratio
       (STWR) and
   *   Lower Oxygen cost of Same Power Output
   *   Improve Post Exercise Recovery Rate (PERR).

When you find yourself in a Nutritional Hole, for God's sake **STOP
DIGGING!**

Key Inflammatory foods to avoid

Sugar- and most food items that convert to sugar quickly, sugar
consumption has increased significantly over the last 200 years.

Americans today typically consume:

* Over 152 pounds of sugar annually
* 200 years ago they consumed about 2 pounds of sugar per year.
* Sugar also goes by other names, such as glucose, lactose, fructose, honey, molasses, fruit juice concentrate and syrup.

Sugar has little nutritional value and also stimulates the immune response, thus elevating C-reactive protein levels, ROS and Inflammation.

Grains -White breads, pastas and rice have been refined to the point that they break down quickly into **sugar** during the digestive process, which can lead to inflammation.

Processed whole-grain products contain gluten, which is a wheat protein. Gluten may contribute to inflammation, especially for individuals who have a gluten sensitivity or celiac disease

Sugar-induced cardiovascular diseases:

Do you consume high amounts of Blatant Sugar or Hidden Sugars?

* If you do then make this note to your diary: there is an association between the consumption of high levels of serum glucose with cardiovascular diseases.

Water, Minerals (electrolytes) and Life

Water is the most abundant constituent of the human body, accounting for one-half to four-fifths of body weight, depending mainly on body fat content. Body water, as a percentage of body mass, is higher in men than in women and tends to fall with age in both.

The normal daily turnover of water is approximately 4% of total body weight in adults and much higher, 15% of total body weight, in infants. Exertion under any of these conditions can cause up to a 10-fold increase in water loss from skin and lungs.

Potassium

The most commonly deficient mineral (not just on low-carb diets) is potassium. *EDR (Estimated Daily Minimum)* for potassium is round 2,000 mg for healthy adults.

Eat food rich in potassium or take supplements (if needed). Be careful about potassium supplements, too much of potassium can be toxic and as dangerous as its deficiency.

AI (Adequate Intake) of potassium is stated to be 4,700 mg a day. There is no upper limit for **healthy individuals** and you shouldn't worry about eating too much of potassium, unless you take supplements.

- **Avocados (~ 1,000 mg per average piece)**
- **Nuts (~ 100-300 mg per 30g / 1 oz serving, depending on the type)**
- **Dark leafy greens (~ 160 mg per cup of raw, 840 mg per cooked)**
- **Salmon (~ 800 mg per average filet)**
- **Mushrooms (~ 100-200 mg per cup)**

Magnesium is commonly deficient in modern diets, including low-carb diets. You should be aware of your intake, especially if you are an active individual like me. RDA for healthy adults is 400 mg a day. However, if you are suffering from magnesium deficiency, you may experience muscle cramps, dizziness and fatigue. Of course, severe magnesium deficiency can result in more serious problems.

Here is a list of foods rich in magnesium:

- Nuts (~ 75 mg per 1 oz of almonds)
- Cacao powder and dark chocolate (~ 80 mg per 1 tbsp cacao powder)
- Artichokes (~ 75 mg per average piece)

- Fish (~ 60 mg per average fillet of salmon)
- Spinach, cooked (~ 75 mg per 1 cup)
- Blackstrap molasses (~ 50 mg per 1 tbsp)

Sodium has always been advised against, especially for those trying to lose weight. The truth is that your body needs extra sodium on a lower-carb diet. The reason is that insulin, which also has the effect of reducing the rate at which sodium is extracted through kidneys, drops and it can cause sodium levels to drop significantly, too.

You should eat 3,000-5,000 mg of additional sodium occurring naturally in food. It's quite simple to get sufficient intake of sodium: Unless you have any medical conditions that restrict your sodium intake, don't be afraid to use salt.

Behavior Modification and Night Time Eating

1. One school of thought is that night time eating can negatively affect our body composition and health as well as increase the likelihood of cardio metabolic issues like diabetes and obesity.
2. The other school of thought on eating before bedtime is it depends on the content and quantity of food consumed.

Discussions in favor of avoiding food before bedtime center on potential negative effects on resting energy expenditure, gastric emptying, and glucose tolerance.

If you must eat before Bedtime:

Although large quantities of food before bedtime may put undue stress on many of our metabolic systems when they should be getting a chance to rest and renew, other evidence suggests that small, nutrient-dense protein based food intake below <200kcals can have a positive effect on recovery.

I do both. On days of catabolic intermittent fasting and long FFA sessions I may stop eating by 6 pm and fast till noon the next day, or on an anabolic day of recovery I may ingest 20g of quality whey protein within an hour before bedtime to help my body repair muscle tissue.

Protein Synthesis, Bedtime Protein and Muscle Recovery

The supply of protein at bedtime on heavy training days may play a pivotal role in performance nutrition as another way to optimize to:

- Achieve improved performance
- Achieve optimal body composition
- Achieve positive metabolic adaptations

Feeding the Specific Need of Workouts and Daily Activities:

Muscle protein synthesis, can be improved when we consume nutrients like protein in before, during, or immediately after exercise. The rule of thumb here is within the 30-90 minute – post workout- window.

There can be a place for Protein intake- prior to sleep

Studies show that compared to people with **NO** nighttime protein ingestion subjects had the following results:

- Whey proteins before sleep produced higher plasma essential amino acid concentrations.
- Increased amino acid concentration translated to a 22% higher muscle protein synthesis rate.
- When combined with exercise training in obese women nighttime did not impact insulin sensitivity.

Sleep and Nutrition

The long and short of pre sleep nutrition data suggest that:

- There may be a metabolic opportunity for active individuals to improve recovery and stimulate muscle protein synthesis with the consumption of a small, high protein- nutrient dense drink before bed (~150 kcals).

The Bottom Line is: Don't Get OLD and FRAIL!

A Sad Environment for Older Individuals

Have you seen all the television advertisements for pharmaceuticals to treat a growing list of chronic conditions? Why not have an equal amount of education like I am trying to convey here, communicated there to the masses?

With people living longer and longer, with more and more identified and advertised- conditions of chronic illness. I see older folks around the independent living facility my mother lives in losing muscle mass and strength at a rapid rate (Sarcopenia). This condition puts these older individuals unnecessarily at risk for accidents- disability, reduced physical performance and an overall -poor quality of life. With this aging and life expectancy are on the rise, we need to address this population with exercise and nutrition such as a little protein at bedtime to maintain/reduce the loss of muscle mass, and even stimulate some growth. **M360** is **NOT** just a high performance program for the young; it is also a life program for anyone at any age who wants to explore optimal metabolic health.

Based on the current available literature, M360 suggest the following:

1. Resistance training and protein ingestion has shown the potential to stimulate muscle growth or synthesis. Most research shows- and it has been our 40-year experience that quality whey protein ingestion (20g) after resistance exercise can stimulate muscle protein synthesis.

2. Daily protein intake in the range of .5–1.0 g protein/lb of lean mass of body weight has shown to provide a positive muscle protein balance, and should be sufficient for most individuals. Protein doses should distributed, every 3–4 h, across the day-with no more than 20-40 grams per setting.
3. The optimal time period during which to ingest protein diminishes with increasing post-exercise time.
4. Again it has been suggested that bedtime- whey protein intake (20–30 g) shows potential to increase overnight Muscle Protein Synthesis MPS and metabolic rate without influencing -overnight- fat burning ability.

During long duration training sessions or events over 90- minute's research suggests the approximately 0.13 g of protein/lb of lean mass-body weight per hour in conjunction with regular carbohydrate intake. These protocols shows promise to suppress excessive muscle damage and improve performance and recovery.

Example: My body weight is 80kg so during training and racing to prevent loss of muscle mass research suggests that I consume 20 grams of Protein per hour of activity.

Protein Feeding Timing

Protein consumption directly after resistance training is a very effective way to improve positive muscle protein balance, which repeated over time, will translate into a positive growth or hypertrophy of muscle.

Post exercise protein consumption should be done- sooner- rather than later, as Muscle Protein Synthesis (MPS) rates peak in the first three (3) hours of post exercise and depending on the intensity of your resistance session can remain elevated for 24–72 h. There is a strong argument that this 24-72 hour window is also cause for slightly increased protein consumption. **Keep in mind single doses of supplemental protein should be no more than 20-40g per serving.**

Key points of Protein feeding

- Protein needs are variable as a result of many personal factors including volume of body composition, total energy intake, exercise, age, and training status. Our range is .5 to 1.5 at the very most in terms of grams per pound of Lean Mass, not Total Weight! Feed the lean, utilize the fat… remember?
- Just as with **TRE** Time Restricted Eating, when and how often we consume protein is important. It is best to spread it across your own personal feed zone. If my feeding window is 10am -6pm I would consume 40 after morning session at 10am then 40 more at 1pm to get my .5 per lean pound. I could add more if by consuming 40 more at 6pm and 20 more grams at bedtime 9pm. That would put me at 140g. protein for a HIGH PROTEIN day for me.

Protein Quality- Selecting a Protein Supplement

- There are 9 essential amino acids (EAA) and 11 non-essential amino acids (NEAAs).
- Our bodies cannot produce 9 essential amino acids so we must consume them in our diet.
- Protein quality referrers to how effective a protein is at promoting Muscle Protein Synthesis (MPS) to promote muscle growth.
- Studies show that products containing animal proteins have the highest % of essential amino acids and do a better job at muscle protein synthesis following resistance training when compared to vegetarian proteins.

Fat Adapted Metabolism and Food

Adiponectin is a protein made by fat cells plays a role in how the body uses sugar, or glucose, and fat for energy. Higher levels of adiponectin are associated with improved sensitivity to insulin and lower blood glucose levels. It can be said that a diet that raises adiponectin levels may be beneficial to improving our Fat Metabolism.

Foods high in Adiponectin:

Avocados

Avocados are the tastiest fats to eat. Having high amounts of potassium, folate and magnesium and being rich in monounsaturated fats, avocados will surely increase your adiponectin levels. Take benefits of avocados as these tasty fats effectively act on your belly fat and help to reduce it.

Olive oil

The polyphenols present in this product helps your body to secrete adiponectin that helps to burn more belly fat as well as regulate the metabolism of fat and sugar. Top your salads with olive oil and lose weight more productively.

Pumpkins and Pumpkin Seeds

Whether you like eating pumpkins or pumpkin seeds – both products are perfect sources to increase adiponectin levels in the body.

Dark Chocolate

Surprised? This tasty food – which is known to make you fat – stimulates the protein that kills your fat. However, there is a small secret. You should eat dark chocolate. Only this kind of chocolate can stimulate adiponectin.

Modify Behavior to include:

1. **Evidence Based Exercise and Physical Activity**
   a. The more you move, the higher fat-burning hormone levels are.

b. Be consistent in your exercises to reach success.

c. Regular exercise/activity is beneficial for those who are fat.

2. **Consume monounsaturated fats**

a. To raise adiponectin levels, replace saturated fats with monounsaturated fats. These can be found in olive oil, avocados and lean beef.

3. **Fish Oil**

a. Fish oil contains beneficial high quality omega-3 that can raise your adiponectin levels. Consider fish oils as part of your daily routine.

b. If your focus is on raising adiponectin in your body, then consuming fish oil is the best option.

4. **Low Dose Aspirin**

a. In addition to its anti-inflammatory properties, aspirin was also observed to increase bleeding time, and later studies demonstrated the utility of aspirin as an antithrombotic agent. Low-dose aspirin regimens around 81 mg/day can effectively suppress platelet aggregation without affecting important endothelial cell functions. The use of a low-dose aspirin regimen as an antithrombotic measure has become increasingly common.

b. Nearly all major heart health organizations have made recommendations regarding aspirin use for CVD prevention, including the AHA/American Stroke Association

c. Extensive review of the literature revealed a strong favor toward the use of low dose aspirin therapy for the primary prevention of CVD.

Functional Nutraceutical Eating to Enhance Performance and Fat Metabolism

Increasing the availability of plasma free fatty acids has been shown to slow the rate of muscle and liver glycogen depletion by promoting the utilization of fat.

Ingested fat, in the form of long-chain triacylglycerols, is largely unavailable during acute exercise, but medium-chain (MCT) triacylglycerols are rapidly absorbed and oxidized.

We have shown that the ingestion of medium-chain triacylglycerols (MCT) in combination with carbohydrate spares muscle carbohydrate stores during 2 h of sub maximal (< 70% VO2 peak) cycling exercise, and improves 40 km time-trial performance.

These data suggest that by combining carbohydrate and medium-chain triacylglycerols as a pre-exercise supplement and as a nutritional supplement during exercise, fat oxidation will be enhanced, and endogenous carbohydrate will be spared.

We have also examined the chronic metabolic adaptations and effects on substrate utilization and endurance performance when athletes ingest a diet that is high in fat (> 70% by energy).

Dietary fat adaptation for a period of at least 2-4 weeks has resulted in a nearly two-fold increase in resistance to fatigue during prolonged, low- to moderate-intensity cycling (< 70% VO2 peak).

Studies suggest that mean cycling 20 km time-trial performance following prolonged sub maximal exercise is enhanced by 80 s after dietary fat adaptation and 3 days of carbohydrate loading.

The relative contribution of fuel substrate to prolonged endurance activity may be modified by training, pre-exercise feeding, habitual diet, or by artificially altering the hormonal milieu or the availability of circulating fuels.

Chronic Disease and the Top 3 Killers of Humans & Diet

The Point of **M360** is to define and execute a Performance Lifestyle to incorporate select components into your day the will reduce and even eliminate Chronic Disease and the TOP 3 Killers of Humankind

1. **Heart Disease**
2. **Cancer**
3. **Respiratory Disease**

In this section we have clearly made the case that diet and nutrition are modifiable risk factors for the development, progression and management of Chronic Disease

- Diet and nutrition are modifiable contributing factors to the development of chronic disease.
- There are increasing volumes of data on the importance of functional food, and the impact- nutraceutical education, can have on the reduction of chronic diseases like: heart disease, cancer and respiratory diseases.

Respiratory Disease -Nutrients -and Breathing Performance

The consumption of potent antioxidants is a major dietary opportunity, to protect us against respiratory disease and the damaging effects of oxidative stress in our airways.

Air pollution and other airborne irritants that trigger inflammatory cell responses can cause excess oxidative stress and ROS. Increased levels of ROS can cause chronic inflammation of our airways.

How can we protect our respiratory system?

The answer once again is a constant dietary intake of antioxidants containing:

- Vitamin C
- Vitamin E
- Flavonoids
- Carotenoids

All of the above compounds are abundantly present in vegetables, and fruits- as well as nuts, chicory, olive oil, avocado oil, cocoa, garlic, dark chocolate and green tea.

Are we consuming enough dietary antioxidants?

The solution to preventing a miserable future of COPD is in our grocery store not in our pharmacy.

Flavonoids

Flavonoids are potent antioxidants that have the ability to neutralize free radical ROS and with it oxidative stress. Flavonoids are widely distributed throughout our diet, with rich sources found in vegetables, fruit, seeds, nuts, roots, dark chocolate, coffee, tea.

M360 is a Functional Whole Foods Approach to Metabolic Fitness

Functional whole foods, offer the benefit of multiple nutraceutical ingredients, including vitamin C, vitamin E, carotenoids and flavonoids.

Target and FEED, your Nutritional Needs with Functional Whole Foods!

In terms of reducing or eliminating Heart Disease, Cancer, Respiratory disease death the research shows it is heavily linked to increasing intake of a plant based diet.

Know your <u>FOOD</u> and what it <u>FEED</u>'s

We live in a **FED** and **UNFED** State. The physical activity levels of our lifestyle dictate our nutritional needs once we identify the components of a productive lifestyle we can tie them all together for a productive sustainable way of life that will lead us away from chronic disease and leave us metabolically healthy. Metabolic fitness for life is our objective.

Here are a list of foods that I call functional foods and their benefits to the activities and lifestyle that we lead.

Number one vegetables, fruits, nuts and seeds, fish and seafood oils herbs spices and condiments.

Chronic disease is brought on by oxidation and inflammation there is a list of foods to protect you against these two villains.

1. **Red Beets**
   a. Beets are an important dietary source of *betaine* and also a good source of folate. The two nutrients work synergistically to reduce potentially toxic levels of *homocysteine*, a naturally occurring amino acid that can be harmful to blood cells therefore contributing to the development of heart disease stroke dementia and peripheral vascular disease beets are also loaded with potassium of file import mineral for heart health data high potassium to sodium ratio which is ideal for human health teacher high magnesium they can be baked boiled or steamed were shredded raw into salads high in calcium iron vitamin a and C great when mixed with a combination of carrots, apples, spinach and, ginger

2. **Broccoli**
   a. Broccoli is vegetable royalty rich in Sulforaphane. Excellent source of anti cancer phytochemicals they neutralize carcinogens the anti cancer properties of broccoli are well established even the American cancer society recommends eating it broccoli is a strong anti oxidant that stimulates detoxification and protects the structure of human DNA broccoli is type two reducing the risk of breast and cervical cancer broccoli is a nutritional powerhouse broccoli is one of the least contaminated foods in terms of pesticide exposure

3. **Carrots**
   a. Carrots have cancer fighting properties and are high in caratanoids- antioxidant compounds found in plants that are

associated with a wide range of health benefits. Caratanoid intake has been associated with a decrease of up to 50% in bladder cervix prostate, colon, larynx and esophageal cancer. Carrots are high in alpha carotene carrots are great for your eyes great sources of lutein. Cooking carrots makes some of the nutrients more by bioavailable.

4. **Kale**

   a. Because kale is a cabbage it actually has even more benefits than its anti-oxidant power alone. Tail contains powerful phytochemicals like cancer fighting indoles, plaque compounds that have been found to have protective effect against breast, cervical, and colon cancer. Kale is high in sulfur which boosts the body's detoxification enzymes and may actually help fight cancer. Kale is loaded with calcium, iron, and vitamins A, C and bone building vitamin K.

5. **Mushrooms**

   a. Shiitake Mushrooms compounds within these mushrooms have immune stimulating effects. Mushrooms in general also contain a powerful anti oxidant which neutralizes dangerous free radicals a few studies have indicated that mushrooms act as metabolic energy enhancers helping to stem lead to break out sugar in red blood cells and help transport fat into the mitochondria of the cells with that can be burned for energy.

6. **Onions**

   a. Onions contain cancer fighting enzymes. In at least two important studies onions help build strong bones. Onions contain a whole pharmacy of compounds with healthy benefits. Onion is one of very selective group of foods that in combination was found to reduce mortality from coronary heart disease by an impressive 20% others included (broccoli, tea, and apples). Some research indicates that onions can help increase the body's production of cancer fighting enzymes like glutathione. Onions contain powerful antioxidants that are anti inflammatory, antibiotic and antiviral they are great source of quercetin, which is a great anti inflammatory compound with beneficial effects on chronic diseases like cancer and heart disease. Quercetin can help relieve asthma in the beaver by blocking some of the inflammatory responses in the airways.

7. **Garlic**

Garlic has been found to have a wide range of medicinal properties ranging from antibacterial to anticancer effects. It has hypolipidemic, antithrombotic and anti-atherosclerotic properties.

*   Garlic can benefit cardiovascular health physical and sexual vitality, cognition and resistance to infection.
*   It also has anti-aging properties raw garlic reduces total cholesterol and LDL low-density lipoprotein while increasing high density lipoprotein HDL garlic as a variety
*   Eating raw garlic daily is associated with significantly reduced risk of prostate colon and stomach cancer
*   In double-blind studies with **garlic** preparations providing a daily dose of at least 10 mg allicin, **blood pressure** readings dropped with typical reductions of 11 mm Hg for the systolic and 5.0 in the diastolic within a 1 to 3-month period.
*   To get enough allicin, **eat** 1 to 4 cloves of **fresh garlic** a day.
*   Many **health** experts consider **garlic** to be a super food due to **its** numerous **health benefits**. ... Unfortunately, cooking **garlic** destroys the **garlic's** ability to make allicin and makes **cooked garlic** generally not as beneficial as raw **garlic**. So chop it up and mix in salads and soups.
*   Each **clove of garlic** contains small amounts of vitamins C, A, E and folate, antioxidants that destroy the free radicals that can damage your cell membranes.

8. **Turmeric**
    a. Slice the root or cut it into pieces and **eat** it by itself, or add it to salads or other fresh dishes. **Turmeric** root has a peppery, slightly bitter flavor and is generally considered safe at doses

of between 1.5 and 3 grams daily, although no minimally effective amount of the root has been established.

a. As a general rule of thumb: **1 inch fresh turmeric = 1 tablespoon freshly grated turmeric = 1 teaspoon ground turmeric**

9. **Granny Smith Apples (An Apple a Day?)**

   a. Apples are full of polyphenols and fiber. Research has identified links between frequent apple consumption and reduced risk of chronic disease. Apples show nutraceutical beneficial effects on our lipid metabolism, vascular function and reduced inflammation

   b. Apples are 2%–3% fiber, including cellulose- with pectin as the major insoluble fiber.

   c. Apple pectin has cholesterol lowering properties and benefits our glucose metabolism.

   d. Apple Juice? Clear apple juice has little polyphenol content. Cloudy apple juice on the other hand contains a good volume of polyphenol due to the lack of the clarification.

   e. In many studies apples have been associated with a reduced risk of coronary heart disease and total cardiovascular disease mortality, as displayed in the Iowa Women's Health Study, where 34,489 subjects free of CVD were followed up for 16 years

   f. Apple fiber, mainly apple pectin, is considered the green apple Nutraceutical responsible for the lowering cholesterol.

   g. The consumption of 2-3 apples per day over a 4 month period was shown to significantly reduce total cholesterols and specifically increased HDL-C.

10. **Ginger**

    a. Anti-oxidative properties of ginger have been tested in many *in vitro* and *in vivo* tests and confirm the antioxidant status of ginger will help to protect us against many chronic diseases.

  b. Ginger has been shown to significantly lower lipid oxidation whilst raising antioxidant enzymes, and serum levels of glutathione.

  c. Ginger is full of health-promoting nutraceuticals shown to:
- Reduce muscle pain
- Reduce angiogenesis
- Improves cardiovascular disorders
- Protect against cancer with functional ingredients like
  1. Gingerols
  2. Shogaol
  3. Paradols
- Improve gastrointestinal health.

11. Avocado's

  a. Avocados introduced to the United States in Santa Barbara, California in 1871

  b. Research data has concluded that consumers of avocado had higher HDL-cholesterol, lower metabolic syndrome, lower weight/BMI, and waist circumference than non-consumers.

  c. Avocado fed diets improved blood lipid profiles- lowering LDL-cholesterol and triglycerides while increasing HDL-c compared to diets without avocado.

  d. Avocados are rich in vitamin A and carotenoids. Absorption is notably higher when avocados are consumed with tomatoes and/or carrots. Holy guacamole!

12. Broth Bone Broth

  a. Bone broth is rich in minerals that support the immune system and contains healing compounds like:
- Collagen
- Glutamine
- The collagen in bone broth heals your gut lining and reduces intestinal inflammation.

13. Chicory Root

  a. Great source of Inulin. Inulin is considered a "prebiotic," promoting healthy bacteria growth in the gut.

NOTE: *Full List of Common Foods we can EAT with Nutraceutical Value at our website: www.metafit.life*

Exercise Nutrition and your BRAIN

More and more evidence suggests that:

- Our Lifestyle, Diet, Activity and ability to Manage Stress is directly linked to delaying the progression many age-related health disorders while improving cognitive function.
- Diet and Exercise is a major consideration in the prevention of neurodegenerative diseases.
- Diet and Exercise are associated with improved cognition and increased brain-derived neurotrophic factor (BDNF), an essential neurotrophin.

Several dietary components have been shown to have a positive effect on our cognitive abilities as we age. Studies show that polyphenols can express a neuroprotective action to suppress neuro-inflammation, and promote cognitive function and memory

Our choice of dietary selections has the power to positively affect multiple brain processes by regulating:

- Neurotransmitter pathways
- Synaptic transmissions
- Membrane fluidity
- Signal-transduction pathways

Nutrition has typically been viewed as carbohydrates, protein and fat macronutrients providing energy and building blocks to our body. We typically do not view our nutrition as a way to prevent and protect us against disease. Nutrition and exercise are **POWERFUL** interventions perfectly capable of reducing negative health effects.

We call it M360 Clinical Fitness because everything we do is targeted at better metabolic health. All the aesthetics of beautiful skin, flat stomachs, and etched physiques are only by- products of sustainable-Metabolic Fitness for Life.

Age Related Gains

Moderate Diet and Exercise can influence our brain morphology as we age. medial temporal lobe and hippocampal volumes are larger in fit adults, indicating that physical activity at any age can increase hippocampal perfusion.

What is the Hippocampus?

The **hippocampus** is the **area** of your **brain** that is associated with motivation, emotion, and memory. A healthy hippocampus is critical to our joy, happiness, and memory to function at an optimal level.

A 1-year randomized controlled trial with 120 older adults (aged 55–80 years), showed that aerobic exercise training increased the size of the anterior hippocampus, leading to improvements in spatial memory. Proper aerobic exercise training along with a diet high in flavonoids is effective at reversing hippocampal volume loss in older adults, which is accompanied by improved memory function.

Everyday Sources Flavonoids

Flavonoids help to protect our body, brain and memory, here are a few represented in six dietary versions:

- Flavones -which are found in celery and parsley
- Flavanones/flavanonols-which are mainly found in herbs, citrus fruit, (oregano), and wine;
- Isoflavones- which are mainly found in soy and soy products;
- Flavonols (e.g. kaempferol, quercetin)- which are found in broccoli, onions, and leeks.

- Flavanols- which are abundant in dark chocolate- green tea, red wine, and
- Anthocyanidins –sources are berry fruits and red wine.

Nutrition and Fatigue

Nutritional interventions can be used to manipulate and reduce fatigue. Fatigue can be defined as an acute impairment of exercise performance, which leads to an inability to produce maximal force output, or power -due to metabolite accumulation or substrate depletion. Fatigue is perceived as the increase in effort necessary to maintain a desired force or power output, and the eventual inability to produce force/power. In a nutshell we lose **Power- Vitality and/or Function.**

Skin Care

After all skin is the biggest organ of the human body and it is on constant 24/7 watch to protect our body from foreign invaders. In addition to keeping it healthy from the inside out with proper nutrition, exercise and stress management it is important to maintenance your skin daily as best you can. Here are a few simple tips:

- **Moisturizers come in several forms** — ointments, creams, and lotions.
  - ○ **Ointments** are mixtures of water in oil, usually either lanolin or petrolatum.
  - ○ **Creams** are preparations of oil in water, which is the main ingredient. Creams must be applied more often than ointments to be most effective.
  - ○ **Lotions** contain powder crystals dissolved in water, again the main ingredient. Because of their high water content, they feel cool on the skin and don't leave the skin feeling greasy. Although they are easy to apply and may be more pleasing than ointments and creams, *lotions don't have the*

same protective qualities. You may need to apply them frequently to relieve the signs and symptoms of dryness.

- **Moisturizers should be used indefinitely** to prevent recurrence of dry skin.
- **Apply moisturizer immediately after washing.** Ointments, creams, and lotions (moisturizers) work by trapping existing moisture in your skin. To trap this much-needed moisture, you need to apply a moisturizer within few minutes of:
  - Drying off after a shower or bath
  - Washing your face or hands

- **Use an ointment or cream rather than a lotion.** Ointments and creams are more effective and less irritating than lotions. Look for a cream or ointment that contains an oil such as olive oil or jojoba oil. Shea butter also works well. Other ingredients that help to soothe dry skin include lactic acid, urea, hyaluronic acid, dimethicone, glycerin, lanolin, mineral oil, and petrolatum.
- **Use only gentle, unscented skin care products.** Some skin care products are too harsh for dry, sensitive skin. When your skin is dry, stop using:
  - Deodorant soaps
  - Skin care products that contain alcohol, fragrance, retinoids, or alpha-hydroxy acid (AHA)
  - Avoiding these products will help your skin retain its natural oils.

Nutrition specific to Skin Health and Aging

Let's face a major common denominator we all share when it comes to taking care of ourselves. In my mind it starts with education. I have said it before and will say it over and over: **"We do not know what we do not know"**.

There is massive POWER in LEARNING. See our Podcast on Skin Health at **Power 2 Learn** on iTunes or Google Play. When it comes to learning and skin care it, of course starts internally and radiates outward. It all starts with learning what your skin as any other organ or cell in your body needs and responds to. What are the specific Nutraceuticals of Optimal Healthy, full functioning, and high performance skin?

Skin Nutrition

Our inner-health and status of aging is said to be reflected in the youthfulness of our skin. Skin has long been reported to reflect our nutritional position. The beauty and skin industry has used flavonoids, polyphenols, and other plant extracts that possess potent anti-oxidant properties for years as topically -oral supplements to improve the appearance of youthful skin.

Beauty comes from the inside

There is a connection between beautiful glowing skin and nutrition. The best prevention strategy against the harmful action of free radicals and skin quality is a well regulated lifestyle:

- Caloric restriction
- General spirit, mind and body care
- Physical exercise
- Lower stress conditions
- Balanced nutritional diet
- Anti-Inflammatory, Anti-oxidative rich food.

The same points we have made through the entire **M360** program are pinpointed with the health of our skin.

Remember: Beauty truly does come from within!

Skin Health and Beauty is a reflection of your metabolism and the health of your being at a cellular level. The mighty mitochondria once again come to your rescue. Help them out by doing what you are doing, seeking the truth and applying your knowledge where it makes sense in your own world.

At this point we have outlined your lifestyle as the organization of the 16 waking hours you have control of each day. You have a choice of physical activity, specific exercise, dietary food selection and options of meditation, relaxation and sleep to recover.

How are you going to put it all together?

By learning you have less and less excuses for poor health and dismal performance.

Optimize the components of your life to optimize your Metabolic Fitness for Life.

Section #3 Summary:

"Feed the Need" says it all! What are we feeding and WHY? Do we feed our Lean Mass (LM) or do we feed our Fat Mass (FM)? Do the foods we eat promote our sugar burning metabolism or our fat burning metabolism? Are we getting more or less fat adapted as an organism?

Do the foods we eat promote Inflammation and Oxidative Stress or do they reduce it?

What is a Functional Whole Food? What is a Nutraceutical? What will a quality plant based diet do for our health? What are Phytonutrients, Flavonoids, Polyphenols, and Sulforaphanes? How can these compounds improve my metabolism, insulin sensitivity and overall performance and healthspan?

What is Autophagy? What is Time Restricted Eating? What is Intermittent Fasting? How can these metabolic activities improve my ATP Production, while reducing ROS?

SECTION #4

Stress Management

Meditation Relaxation & Concentration

LIFESTYLE COMPONENT #4

Stress Management

Life is one continuous cycle of Load and Recover Stress Dynamics. Our **"Stress Response"** is critical to the affect stress has on our performance and healthspan.

How do you respond to STRESS?

We would be remiss to leave this section out of our book. The ability to relax, concentrate & recover is critical to the sustained execution of the components of your **NEW** lifestyle and the absolute requirement of your optimal flow of energy.

Concentration, Relaxation, Recovery and Meditation is like an exercise- you can do it anywhere anytime to get yourself psychologically centered into a positive winning mindset.

Power 2 Learn is personal power to motivate and re-motivate your mind- to address life with a new variety of sustainable options.

- Understanding your metabolism, how it works and how you can help your mitochondria do what they do- while minimizing inflammation and over oxidation.

- It all starts and ends with a winning mindset capable of self motivation, the ability to relax under pressure and to meditate and recover.

These are learned components of **PERSONAL POWER** in your arsenal to deal with split second decisions in life.

If you have read and participated in our workbook, while taking time to listen to a few podcast episodes while you gently walk, hike, jog, run, swim, ride or paddle, then you have grown. You have empowered the cells of your body; you are altering your Mindset.

You are winning!

Each day brings a new opportunity to learn and with it a canvas to MASTER your LIFESTYLE; however you must first master your mindset. Here is the definition:

Dictionary.com definition of Mindset says it all:

> *"A fixed mental attitude or disposition that predetermines a Person's responses to and interpretations of situations"*

How is your Current Mindset Working for YOU? _____

It is never too late to change your state of mind; you can do it right **NOW!** It sounds trite but it is true, the glass is half full- **NOT** half empty. As a reader and listener of our programs, you are winning.

- You are **WINNING** because you are **LEARNING,** and you are learning because you are **SEEKING. NEVER STOP SEEKING TO LEARN!**

It is not hard to understand that by changing the components of your lifestyle, by reducing inflammation as measured by hs-CRP levels, whilst lowering free radical oxidation (ROS) you can dramatically improve your metabolic fitness for life.

You should find all this new empowerment enlightening, which in itself will improve your awareness and mindset.

- Take tiny manageable steps.
- Give yourself credit for each winning stroke of your own personal program.
- Keep seeking and asking better and better questions.
- Keep learning and you will be able to sustain metabolic fitness for life!

What is Stress?

Stress is:

"Any uncomfortable emotional experience, accompanied by Predictable, biochemical, physiological and behavioral changes"

Stress affects us all, regardless of gender, circumstance, or race. Stress will have a massive detrimental effect on our metabolism and our life, our mindset, and our physiology, if we let it.

Stress can be a beneficial tool at producing- a boost of energy to get us through situations like exams, deadlines, life situations and competitions. It is extreme- chronic amounts of stress that will inflict chronic conditions and adversely affect our immune, cardiovascular, and central nervous systems.

Stress can harm our health

Extreme stress can destroy our health. Constant excessive stress, that persists over a prolonged period of time is physically and psychologically debilitating. Unchecked stress left unchecked will increase cellular inflammation which will cascade into oxidative stress (OS) ultimately finding a home in chronic disease. Don't let this happen! We can prevent this, or at least slow the monster down.

Do you let silent- chronic levels, of stress grind at you day in and day out?

Untreated chronic stress can lead to a number of serious health conditions such as:

- **Anxiety**
- **Insomnia**
- **Muscle pain**
- **High blood pressure**
- **Weakened immune system**
- **Digestive issues**

Research shows that stress contributes to the development of major illnesses, such as:

- **Chronic Disease**
- **Depression**
- **Obesity**

Unhealthy chronic stress management, such as **"overeating of comfort"** foods, is directly contributing to our obesity epidemic.

According to the American Psychology Association (APA), over 60% of Americans report that personal health concerns, or health problems affecting their family as the primary source of stress. Yet, in spite of this concern, over 33% of Americans never discuss ways to manage stress with their healthcare provider.

Our response to everyday chronic stress is often ignored and poorly managed, as well as our exposure to traumatic events. Consequences of chronic stress can be very serious, specifically as it contributes to anxiety and depression.

Those of us who suffer from anxiety and/or depression have twice the proclivity toward developing cardiovascular disease those without.

Studies indicate there is a strong association between suffering from chronic stress and indulging in self medicating addictive substance abuse.

Are <u>YOU</u> managing your stress?

According to many studies- chronic stress is directly related to insomnia with more than 40% of all adults revealing that they lie awake at night because of stress.

It is critical that we do our best to go to bed at the same time each night with the objective to get 8-quality hours of sleep.

Remember the answer to the question: What is the most important part of each 24 hour segment of your life? SLEEP... Quality Sleep!

Again it is very important that you take a look at your sleep environment and turn off all the lights and noise you possibly can to make your room cool and inviting for quality 8 hour sleep cycle. Make the appropriate lifestyle changes to reduce stress and ultimately prevent health problems.

M360 wants you to consider simplifying your life by immersing yourself into and defining what you do with the 16 waking hours you are blessed with each day.

As we discussed in Section 1: What are the components of your day?

This is your lifestyle! Consider integrating 4-new components into your 16 hour day.

- With a little effort you can improve your lifestyle, and modify your behavioral choices- reach out NOW and take the essential steps that are available to you to optimize overall health, and avoid chronic stress which leads to chronic disease.

- Mastering your Lifestyle is simply mastering quality components of your day to work for you- rather than against you.

At the baseline, these selected components must support optimal metabolic function, be sustainable and motivate your mindset!

Learn to recognize and change behaviors that cause stress.

We know it is not easy, but you can do it and it is worth it in spades as you age.

- Take little steps like adding a daily walk to your schedule. Walks will reduce your stress, improve your emotional health, and benefit metabolic fat adaptation as well as free your mind.
- Being active and becoming better aware of the components of your lifestyle and **HOW** you metabolically respond to people, places, and things, is a small but powerful change you can make to manage stress.

It can all sound so scientific and complicated, yet when you boil it all down it is very simple. The purpose of learning is not to go around spewing a lot of technical terms, it is to improve your baseline understanding of **WHY** you need to **ACT,** and **ACT NOW**- on certain simple **COMPONENTS** you must take the time to **DEFINE** and **IMPROVE**.

Enjoy a Life of Evidence Based Physical Activity and Nutrition

Feel-good, moderate intensity physical activity, increases our production of endorphins. Endorphins are neurotransmitters in our brain that reduce anxiety and depression.

It is for this reason that the exercise component of **M360** is driven in a **FEEL GOOD ZONE** of intensity designed to **STIMULATE** not over-stress and destroy. The days of No Pain- No Gain are over my friend, we are smarter than that, because we have **LEARNED!**

Remember:

High levels of chronic stress, over a prolonged period of time, can result in- bouts of anxiety and depression. If this condition persists, it should be shared with a licensed mental health professional, such as a psychologist.

Research shows that chronic stress can be improved with interventions such as lifestyle change, nutraceutical adaptations, and in some situations, medication. There is a time and place for medication as long as we do **NOT** abuse it, only to make things worse in the long-term.

A psychologist can help you overcome the barriers that are stopping you from living a healthy life, manage stress effectively and help identify behaviors and situations that are contributing to your consistently high stress level.

When we are stressed our body is designed to?

Stress is actually designed to be an asset to our metabolism.

- Stress is designed to speed up our heart rate and divert blood away from our gut and in our muscle cell so we can run away from danger.
- Stress will constrict the pupils of our eyes to confront attackers.
- Stress will dilate our lungs and increase oxygenation of our blood, to stimulate the metabolic conversion of stored energy in our liver into ATP fuel for stamina and strength..
- Optimal **STRESS RESPONSE** is designed to keep us safe.

When we are stressed the hypothalamus of our brain makes a hormone called Corticotrophin-Releasing Hormone. If we allow ourselves to bath in this STRESS SOUP of nerve chemicals and hormones too long, we will impair our immune system.

Stress hormones stimulate our adrenal glands to release a hormone called cortisol. The exogenous prescribed version of cortisol is called Cortisone, which is considered one of the most powerful anti-inflammatory drugs available today.

When we are stressed- our body is basically giving itself metabolic shots of this endogenous version of cortisone (cortisol). Although this hormone works wonderfully as a powerful anti-inflammatory it can also dial down our immune system's ability to fight infection.

We must better understand our stress response:

Chronic activation of our hormonal system can be a problem to our health!

Studies find that 25% of Americans are experiencing high levels of stress (rating their stress level as 8 or more on a 10-point scale), with another 50% reporting moderate levels of stress (a score of 4 to 7).

We are engulfed in a world of chronic stress looming work issues, family issues, chronic bombardment of instantaneous news, good, bad, and ugly- all have a persistent physiological effect that can trigger a cascade of stress hormones, producing a orchestrated chain reaction of physiological and psychological change.

Chronic stress to any situation can be very unpleasant. Chronic stress elevates our resting heart rate and is detrimental to our heart rate variability (HRV). With advances in technology we can now readily track these biometrics and see the 30,000 ft vie of cause and effect. We can start to eliminate unnecessary beats of the heart and gasp's for air, while reducing muscle tension and undue sweat. In nutshell we can learn to better deal with stress and manage this life altering response to people places and things. We no longer have to be slaves to our own lack of knowledge or ignorance!

Our Response to stress can be: "Fight or Flight"

"Fight-or-Flight" response is a survival mechanism that enables us to react quickly to life-threatening situations. This hormonal sequence of events prepares us to **fight off** –or- **flee from** perceived threat.

We tend to overreact to stress that is **NOT** life-threatening, such as family issues, work drama, social irritants and self inflicted pressure. Perhaps our greatest tool is to learn how to let go, learn to EXHALE and let it be.

Modern research- at the time of this writing, have gained new insight into the long-term effects chronic stress, the consensus is simple-repeated-chronic- activation of our stress response takes a toll on the body. This "Toll on the Body" is in most cases, is unnecessary with the correction starting with better self-awareness.

Studies teach us that chronic stress contributes to:

- High blood pressure
- Promotes the formation of oxidized LDL and artery-clogging deposits
- Causes brain changes that may contribute to
  - **Anxiety**
  - **Depression**
  - **Addiction**

Chronic stress can contribute to obesity via:

1. Direct actions such as emotional – over eating.
2. Indirect actions such as poor sleep and lack of exercise.

How do you filter life? Alarm or <u>FALSE</u> Alarm or ...

Our brain via the nervous system it controls governs all stress. When we confront self perceived stress- in any form, our nervous system goes to work- which can be good or bad. Learning again **LEARNING** is the key to how we **FILTER** our response to what crosses the path of our life. Using our ability to **THINK**, our **THOUGHTS** can prevent false alarm as we learn what **NOT** to react to.

How are YOU reacting to LIFE?

Our self perception, ability to reason and think can help us to filter out unnecessary chronic stress and better control our autonomic nervous system (ANS) response. Our ANS controls involuntary body functions as:

- Heartbeat/Heart Rate
- Blood pressure
- Breathing
- Dilation/Constriction of blood vessels and small airways

The autonomic nervous system has two components we focus on at M360:

1. The **sympathetic** nervous system. **Drives Metabolism Up**.
2. The **parasympathetic** nervous system. **Drives Metabolism Down**.

The sympathetic nervous system (SNS) is the **GO** button. **OUR SNS triggers the fight-or-flight response.** The parasympathetic nervous system is the "dial down knob", cannot turn it off we do that when we die, but we can learn to **TURN DOWN THE VOLUME!!**

Note: for these simple reasons we never promote exercise late at night, or eating a high caloric load of food before bedtime. This is the time of day we should be de-activating the sympathetic nervous system, and activating the parasympathetic nervous system.

Our parasympathetic nervous system (PNS) up regulates our ability to **"rest and digest"**. Our PNS response system- calms our body down.

Learning new tools and arming ourselves with real methods- to activate and deactivate it are the key to our successful, and sustainable- ability to manage stress.

There are many **FEEL GOOD** ways we will **LEARN** to do this. Athlete or not it is a critical tool to be able to ramp yourself up for a presentation, or competition as well as dial yourself down- to better recover and respond to the next stimulus you will need to see your goals through to fruition over time.

At **M360** we feel it is important to bring these concepts into our Lifestyle through Exercise and Physical Activities. The more aware we are of how it feels to stimulate and recover the better we can learn to deal with both **activation** and **deactivation** of our **Autonomic Nervous System (ANS)**.

The more **AWARE** you are of what it **FEELS** like to drive your heart rate from 60% of your MHR to 80% of your MHR and back to 60% MHR -the better you will become at recognizing and addressing **STRESS**.

Our ability to recover, or improve post exercise recovery rate (PERR) stems not only from Physical Fitness, but also from the Psychological ability to RELAX, CONCENTRATE and DE-ACTIVATE the sympathetic response by ACTIVATION of the parasympathetic system. I call it ANS (autonomic nervous system) Fitness.

What is your ANS Fitness?

The Process of STRESS

1. The amygdala portion of our brain sends a signal to the hypothalamus which activates the sympathetic nervous system

through our autonomic nerves to our adrenal glands. **BAM...**
Game ON!

2. Our body responds to this activation of our sympathetic nervous system by pumping the hormone epinephrine (also known as adrenaline) into our bloodstream.

3. Epinephrine/Adrenaline circulating in our bloodstream brings about a slew of physiological changes.

    a. Our heart rate increases pushing higher volumes of blood into our:
        i. Muscles
        ii. Heart
        iii. Other vital organs
    b. Our blood pressure go up
    c. Our rate of breathing goes up
    d. Airways in our lungs dilate to wide open. Oxygen consumption per breathe along with our STATE of ALERTNESS is maximized..
    e. Hearing and sight become sharper.
    f. Epinephrine/Adrenaline also triggers the **release of blood sugar** (glucose) and fats from the storage sites of our body.
    g. Substrates become **ATP Energy** to fund the **Fight** or the **Flight.**

Metabolic changes listed above, as a response to **STRESS** or perceived stress, are- for the most part- instantaneous. The stress response is great if there is an actual threat, but in the world we live in it becomes smudged line of low level chronic activation that over activates cortisol, insulin and blood sugar and metabolic issue begin to increase inflammation and oxidative stress.

What are our techniques to counter chronic stress?

When we cannot find a way to put the brakes on and dial down stress, chronic low-levels of stress stay activated. Picture pulling into your driveway and turning off the key, yet your engine continues to rev just above idling. These scenarios will prematurely destroy our car and it is **NO** different with our health. Hello oxidation -inflammation and the cascade of situations and chronic conditions that can lead to Chronic Disease!

Are you starting to see the Simplistic Components within the Complex Maze?

- Consistent surges of epinephrine/adrenaline- as a response to stress can damage blood vessels, raise blood pressure and increase the risk of heart attacks and strokes. Oh and guess what? Increase O/S and with it potential oxidation of LDL and we back in a bad sequence of events.
- Fortunately, we can learn techniques to counter the stress response, and with it the nasty cascade of events that lead us down a dark road.

Meaningful ways we can activate our Relaxation response

Learning how to execute and counter a stress response can be as simple as replacing it with a **RELAXATION RESPONSE.** Here are a combination of fun, and meaningful approaches, that elicit the relaxation response:

- Deep relaxed- abdominal belly breathing and learning to exhale
- Mindful focus on a soothing words (such as peace or calm, serenity)
- Visualization of tranquil scenes
- Repetitive Mantra or Prayer
- Yoga
- Stretching
- Tai chi
- Dry Brushing
- Warm Baths
- Relaxing Naps

- Barefoot Walks (Grounding)
- Playing Musical Instruments
- Painting for fun
- Gardening
- Loving Pets and Nature

Mindful states- of willing relaxation, with a focus on breathing (exhaling), conducted with an attitude of focus and release have been shown to work at reducing stress and with it all the nasty side effects. These techniques are certainly worthy of our consideration of employment into our lives.

Research is conclusive that-people who practiced the relaxation response- had significant reductions in systolic blood pressure. and reduced levels of blood pressure.

- Once again, why not seek these types of natural remedies to chronic conditions rather than just automatically throw pharmaceuticals at every issue?

Physical activity

Physical activity can be utilized as a tool to stifle our buildup of stress in several ways.

- Walk when you fee stressed
- Deepen your breathing with a focus on exhalation
- Drop a few yoga sequences
- Glide into a few tai chi movements
- Ease into a few relaxing stretches
- Think a mental and physical state/mindset of calm.

Walking

Walking at a brisk pace provides a natural bipedal pumping action which helps to move lymph through our **lymphatic system**. Our lymphatic **system** has no pump, so walking is a great way to give it a manual push. Our circulatory **system** has a heart to pump blood, whilst our lymphatic depends on movement to assist the flow of bodily fluid.

Learn to enjoy simple movements to reduce lymphatic pooling by using low-level active recovery activities such as walking and biking. The active muscle contractions place pressure on the passive veins and lymphatic vessels to push fluid back into central circulation. Walking slowly for a few minutes each day is a great way to amplify recovery.

Dry Brushing

Our skin is our largest organ, and there is one simple step you can add to your pre shower routine that can dramatically improve skin condition– dry skin brushing!

The benefits of dry skin brushing go beyond skin deep aesthetics; dry brushing offers total body benefits to our overall health.

Dry skin brushing gently removes dead skin cells- leaving you feeling invigorated and relaxed. Dry brushing also activates the removal of waste via our lymphatic system. Dry skin brushing offers multiple benefits including:

1. **Stimulate Your Lymphatic System**
2. **Exfoliation**
3. **Increase Circulation**
4. **Stress Relief relaxation response**
5. **Improve Digestion**
6. **It's Invigorating**

Get a high-quality dry brush made from natural materials, one with bristles that feel stiff, but not too stiff. Get one with a long handle so you can get your entire back.

Dry brushing can be done multiple times daily. Brushing is best done on dry skin before you shower. I do it before my morning shower and before my evening bath and I sleep like a baby. I also do it on occasion if I feel stressed to relax before a stretch or walk.

When brushing, for circulation and lymphatic system- always brush toward your heart. Start with the soles of your feet, working your way up your leg's- to your arms, chest, back, and stomach, to include your entire body.

The pressure you apply while brushing your skin should be firm but not painful use a one way stroking movement. Your skin should be pink after a session and you can brush for as long (or as little) as you'd like. An average dry brushing session may last between two and 20 minutes. Stimulate don't Destroy!

Grounding

Grounding, also referred to as earthing is walking barefoot in clean grass or sand. Research indicates it helps to relax us and reduce pain, yet another way to activate our relaxation response. We did this when I ran track and field at the University of Arizona after a hard track session we would do barefoot strides for relaxation, warm down and foot flexibility/strength. Never underestimate the importance of your feet.

Grounding has been proven to relieve pain as well as reduce various chemical factors related to inflammation. My experience and research show us that sustained contact with good ole Mother Earth can have sustained benefits. Spend some Relaxing Time- Bare Foot.

Hot Baths (Hydrotherapy) Thermal Medicine

The use of water therapy/hydrotherapy is as old as man. Hot Springs and Thermal Medicine are important rituals of relaxation, with multiple roots- to a diverse variety of cultures around the world. Use of hot, cold and frozen water has produced undeniable benefits in a number of situations, over time.

Vasodilatation via hot water therapy and low temperature sauna bathing (LTSB) at 140°F for 15-30 min improves cardiac function.

Soothing warm water triggers our skin to release endorphins stimulating a cascade of relaxation responses right down to lowering inflammation cellular oxidative stress.

Research indicates that spending time in a sauna or hot bath around 105 -108 °F can:

- Reduce the risk of heart attack
- Improve blood sugar control
- Lower blood pressure

General States of Focus, Relaxation and Mindfulness

Tai chi is a gentle way to fight stress and improve mindfulness

> **"Tai chi helps reduce stress and anxiety and helps increase flexibility and balance".** -Mayo Clinic

What is Tai Chi

Tai chi is an ancient Chinese tradition we practice as a graceful form of exercise.

Slow, focused movements performed in harmony with deep breathing that coincides with a variety of specific movements.

Tai chi, also referred to as tai chi chuan, is a gentle- noncompetitive-physical flow of movement and stretching. Tai chi is a flow of postures-one into the next without pause, to maintain a constant fluid motion in sync with deep- relaxed breathing..

Tai chi can best be described as Mindful Movement. We incorporate a sequence of mindful-movement into daily sessions of M360 to bring general awareness to the totality, fluidity of our body, our being, our general perception of balance in **ALL** activities.

Why try tai chi?

Regular execution of tai chi can be a positive part of our overall approach to improving your health. Benefits of Tai chi include:

- Dramatically improve Spatial IQ (space awareness)
- Decreased stress, anxiety and depression
- Improved mood
- Improved aerobic capacity
- Increased energy and stamina
- Improved flexibility, balance and agility
- Improved muscle strength and definition

Research suggests that tai chi may also help:

- Enhance quality of sleep
- Enhance the immune system
- Help lower blood pressure
- Improve joint pain
- Improve symptoms of congestive heart failure
- Improve overall well-being
- Reduce risk of falls in older adults

Mindful Stretching

At M360 we perform 3 types of stretching:

1. Static Stretching to relax improve general range of motion (ROM)
2. Dynamic Stretching to prepare muscle for activity
3. Proprioceptive Neuromuscular Stretching (PNF) done in pairs

Swimming (Fitness and Hydrotherapy)

I cannot say enough about swimming and all the benefits of being weightless, suspended in a body of water. Swimming can improve strength, lung capacity, flexibility, decrease tension improve mood and overall general wellness.

Cool Bedroom Sleeping Environment

Heat will increase wakefulness and decrease slow wave -and rapid eye movement (REM) modes of sleep.

Cooler temperatures do the opposite and promote deeper sleep with full cycles of slow wave and REM sleep.

The temperature of the room in which you sleep, is referred to as your thermal environment which can dramatically affect the mechanisms that regulate the quality of our sleep.

Remember the forward to this book?

What is the most important part of our day?

Sleep is the answer, and a consistent patter n off sleep-wake rhythm that is repeated each 24-hour cycle. Our core temperature flow slightly up and down as we sleep, increasing during the waking phase and decreasing during deeper renewing phases.

- It is critical that we establish a consistent pattern of our own sleep-wake rhythm. This is our own personal circadian rhythm which is important for maintaining quality recovery sleep.

Social support- metafit.life group support by like minded friends

Confidants, friends, acquaintances, and companions can all provide a life-enhancing social net — that may increase our longevity. People in general- who enjoy close relationships receive emotional support that indirectly helps us in times of chronic stress and/or crisis. Our social net can provide the **"assurance"** that we are **NOT** alone in our journey, bringing some comfort that allows us to relax a little bit more.

Our **M360 Fitness Clinics** draw like minded people. People who are interested in success, seekers-who monitor and track evidence based metrics that define and **PROVE** our progress. There is enormous **Personal Power** among successful people when they learn to collaborate and forge a powerful sense of camaraderie. Our group accountability is what drives the essence of our **SUCCESS!**

The POWER of Breathing to release and deactivate stress response

There are plenty of ways to relieve stress:

1. Proper "Feel Good M360 Exercise"
2. 15-30 minute soaks in a 105-108°F hot bath
3. Dry brushing
4. Walking
5. Swimming
6. Mindful Stretching/Yoga
7. Massage

Without even thinking about it, something you are doing right now is the most powerful stress reliever of all:

BREATHING!

As we have already discussed in previous sections- deep breathing is not only relaxing, it is scientifically proven to affect:

- Heart function
- Brain function
- Digestion
- Our immune system
- Even the epigenetic expression of genes
- As well as simple State of Relaxation

Putting On the Stress Brake

Breathing exercises can have immediate effect on our body by altering:

- Blood ph
- Lower blood pressure
- Improving HRV (variability of heart rate)

Mastering our awareness and pattern of breathing can train our body's reaction to stressful situations and reduce the production of harmful stress hormones.

- Rapid breathing is monitored and driven by our **sympathetic** nervous system (SNS). SNS is part of the *"fight or flight"* response — the part activated by stress.
- Deep breathing with a focus on EXHALATION stimulates the opposing **parasympathetic nervous system (PNS)** reaction — the one that *calms us down.*

Remember the cover of this book: Mastering Your Lifestyle?

It starts with mastering your awareness and control of breathing. So simple yet so overlooked. Try it right now; try altering your **"State"** with a few relaxing belly breaths initiated with a **"Voluminous"** sign of exhalation.

Our **"relaxation response"** is controlled by our **Vagus Nerve**. Think of us racing down a highway at 100 miles an hour. Dangerous speeding is our stress response, and our Vagus Nerve is the brake pedal.

When we get stressed and have our gas pedal to the floor- we need to learn how to take deep- slow breaths, and engage our stress brake. Awareness is the key to being able to mentally observe our own response to a variety of situations and exercise control over our own stress response to people, places and things. Is it too simple to say that it starts with a thought and a breath?

Learning to apply the brake and deactivate the sympathetic and activate the parasympathetic nervous system is a POWER TOOL you can adopt now!

Changing our Gene Expression and Metabolic Outcome (Epigenetics)

Harvard researcher Herbert Benson coined the term "The Relaxation Response" in 1975 with a book of the same name. The writing showed that meditation, using breathing as a center of focus, can alter our stress response.

Research shows that breathing can alter the basic activity of your cells, and even change our expression of genes (epigenetics). Never underestimate the power of breathing and the application of your mind!

We can use our mind to change our body, and the expressions of genes we are changing are the genes responding to stress. Remove the stress and with it the stress response or gene expression.

How is Our MIND directing Our BODY?

Breathing is obviously very important, but it is NOT the answer to every issue. However, holding a better awareness to the POWER of our breath is both a wise and prudent thought to establish within your components of life. Deep mindful breathing and self awareness is our starting point, our window into our own metabolic health and metabolic reaction to LIFE!

The best part our breathing component it the fact it is free, and literally-right under our nose and **WE** can activate them **NOW!**

Can stress management lower inflammation and improve health?

Metafit.life M360 is focused on optimizing your health by first reducing your levels of Inflammation and Oxidation as measurable by the very important Biomarker of hs-CRP.

Inflammation and Oxidation, as we now know- is a robust and reliable predictor of all-cause mortality. Proinflammatory conditions and C-reactive protein (CRP) play a role in:

- Cardiovascular disease
- Type II diabetes
- Arthritis
- Osteoporosis
- Alzheimer's disease
- Periodontal disease Frailty
- Functional decline

There is strong evidence that inflammation influences tumor cell proliferation, and angiogenesis. Modern science now considers inflammation a risk factor for most cancer.

Lifestyle choices can substantially increase or decrease inflammation!

Behavior Induced Inflammation and Oxidation

In addition to exercise and obesity, **anxiety** and **depressive symptoms** can raise pro-inflammatory conditions. Behavior and thought affects inflammation, and can directly provoke increases in pro-inflammatory conditions throughout our body. Even modest levels of psychological stress have been linked to the sustained —overproduction- of inflammation and oxidation.

Mindful stretching and Yoga

Yoga has a reputation for stress reduction. Many studies suggest that yoga reduces symptoms of anxiety and depression.

Yoga- in conjunction with deep breathing-, with a focus on release, is a great way to deactivate our sympathetic nervous system, and activate vagal-parasympathetic activity; both have a positive effect on our immune system, and lower inflammation levels.

As we adopt some of the methods in this section, from dry brushing to Yoga we can begin to develop the ability to minimize autonomic and inflammatory responses in stressful situations.

Can we reduce inflammation and stress with attitude and breathing?

Emotional and physical stressors activate immune and enhance endogenous- proinflammatory production.

A recent study suggested that regular yoga practice can reduce inflammation, improve cardiorespiratory fitness, and reduce symptoms of anxiety and depression.

Further studies show that 20 minutes of Tai Chi Chih, described as "meditation through movement," was very effective in reducing sympathetic activity, compared to passive rest.

Stress management as we view it at **M360** is developing the awareness and power to minimize autonomic and inflammatory responses to stressful encounters. This will reduce the influence and burden that stress has on us.

Learning to Relax, Concentrate & Exhale:

Training the mind is much different than most people imagine it to be. In a nutshell people try too hard to achieve some sort of Nirvana, fall short and quit trying. This is often the product of Too Much Expectation.

Don't let expectations get in the way of process! Most people think they have to stop thoughts or eliminate feelings and emotions, to get into some higher state, but that will only get in your way. The easiest way to think of active meditation is to picture clouds in a blue sky just drifting by, like the thoughts and feelings drift through your mind. Let them go, relax, use your power to exhale and bring your attention to your breathing. I would add a smile; it is amazing what a smile will do. Improving your mindset is about learning to change your relationship with thoughts and feelings. Just like the entire point of this book is for you to change your relationship with your lifestyle, diet, exercise, and activity. Learn new ways of dealing with minute to minute choices. Smile instead of frowning, eat a nutritious food rather than submit to a craving. Respect yourself, rather than walk around loathing you decisions. As you gain perspective on your lifestyle and it's components you will naturally gain a stronger sense of calm. This is what I would refer to as becoming empowered to get more out of life.

Focus on tangible components of your lifestyle you have right in front of you, RIGHT NOW. Remember the podcast and section 3 on breathing?

Do we utilize the Power of Breathing
In our Day –to- Day Quest for Better Health?

The power of exhaling exercises to lower inflammation:

Try a simple yoga breathing exercise for as little as a minute a day to reduce stress and relax. It's best to pick a regular time to practice yoga breathing, whether it's first thing in the morning, when you transition from work to home, or right before bedtime.

1. Come to a comfortable seat and sit upright with your spine tall.
2. Close your eyes and bring your attention to your natural breath.
3. Inhale through your nostrils for four counts and imagine your lungs filling up from the bottom, middle, and all the way to the top.

4. Exhale through your nostril for four counts. Imagine your lungs emptying from top, middle, and the bottom.
5. Repeat this breath pattern for 10 cycles.
6. Next, inhale your nostrils for four counts, hold for four counts, and then exhale through your nostrils for four counts.
7. Repeat this breath pattern for 10 cycles.

Motivation

What drives you? What inspires you? Everything we have covered in this program is worthless unless you are willing and driven to adopt and execute a few of the principles we have discussed. Just a few simple-permanent changes can alter your health for life.

Motivation defined

Motivation is defined as the

"Energizing of Behavior in Pursuit of a Goal"

Motivation is a fundamental component of our interaction with the world and with each other. Animals share motivation to obtain basic needs, including food, water, sex and social interaction. Meeting these needs is a requirement for survival, as humans we must channel our motivation in appropriate quantities and at appropriate times. Our motivational drive must be adapted to our internal state as well as external environmental conditions. We have options and social avenues to execute them within our society.

What are your options and how to you execute them currently?

Stress Management and Motivation

The ability to pick and choose your battles is very important to your level of motivation. You must first **"CHOOSE"** to pursue success by learning all you can about what your options are. WHY is a huge word and will certainly drive or kill long term motivation.

Why do we do what we do?

Show me the WHY and then we can discuss WHAT it is we specifically NEED or WANT to do!

I have learned that rest and relaxation is a critical part of my program. Rest and relaxation bring about focus, clarity, recovery and the ability to execute my chosen lifestyle components long term. It is only in the long term mindset that we truly affect meaningful outcomes.

I want you to start viewing your hot bath or your stretching/yoga/ meditation time as a daily exercise. Choose your own individual routine to fits your lifestyle. Make elements of this section of the book permanent components of your lifestyle.

My own personal example that I have found extremely valuable is each night after I have executed all of the chosen components of my lifestyle I take time to Dry Brush my body for 2-5 minutes followed by a 105 degree hot bath for 15-20 minutes and off to bed. This has an enormous affect on my sleep pattern, feels great and puts me in a state of success to achieve at every level, by setting up conditions of deeper sleep and proper recovery to face the next day and be at my best.

What Does <u>YOUR</u> Personality and Attitude PROJECT?

What are the intrinsic natures or indispensable qualities and character that determine the essence of who you are?

People project a broad spectrum of ESSENCE. The very word is very near and dear to me. I cannot speak for you the reader or listener, but I can see and feel the essence of other people. Positive and Negative essence draws me in or drives me away. I have learned the power of surrounding yourself with positive people who are riddled with the positive intrinsic nature and drive to succeed, to learn to perform and to improve. People who want to **WIN**! People who can take a loss, but use lose as fuel to persist and succeed and what drives them.

Do we <u>WANT</u> Success? What is Success?

Success in life can be defined either objectively or subjectively.

- Objective success is doing well according to some common metric uniformly applied to all individuals in a society.
- Subjective success concerns an individual's personal assessment of his or her life situation.

Which matters more: how we stack up to others according to widely held standards or, rather, how we think and feel about our own lives?

How we frame this question is critical to how we feed our essence and drive to achieve and accomplish a variety of objectives. Changing the metabolic landscape of our bodies starts with a check up from the neck up and adopting winning behavior to drive our evidence based program across all 4 sections of this book: Lifestyle-Exercise-Diet-Stress Management.

Successful People

Successful People are resilient people, who use positive attitudes & emotions to rebound from, and find positive meaning in, stressful encounters. We must be:

- Persistent
- Resilient
- Determined to Succeed

We must realize there will be setbacks and imperfections in our lives that we must press up against, embrace and navigate around or through.

Napoleon was said to "Blow up his Ships" upon landing to make a statement there is only one way forward… **WIN!** There is **NO GOING BACK!**

Successful Individuals "bounce back" from negative events effectively, whereas others get caught in a rut, unable to get out of their own negative mindset.

We must develop the ability to move on despite negative stressors and demonstrate the winning concept known as resilience.

Psychological resilience refers to effective coping and adaptation although faced with loss, hardship, or adversity.

Are <u>YOU</u> Psychologically Resilient?

Resilient individuals have optimistic, zestful, and energetic approaches to life, are curious and open to new experiences, and are characterized by a high level of positive emotionality. What it all comes down to is having the right attitude and making the effort in the right direction to bring about a positive sustainable change.

Execute your Intelligence

We **MUST** Execute what we learn and never ever stop the motivation to learn! We must <u>**BE ON FIRE**</u> with desire to improve- with a never ending hunger to learn!

Global Accountability to Baseline Bio-Metrics

We must also be accountable and track our metrics over time to help us learn more about our own reaction to people, places and things. I use a Garmin Fenix 5 to track my walks, paddles, rides, swims, M360 sessions, Zwift competitions, epic events like the Olympic Training Center indoor 24 hour ride and the general ebb and flow of load and recover stress and recovery in terms of Resting Heart Rate (RHR) and Heart Rate

Variability (HRV). I call it the 30,000 ft view of our lifestyle. You cannot see it in 1 Day it is a pattern or trend you see over Months and Years.

We are dealers of Garmin for the very reason that we request each member to purchase a quality Garmin Personal Device to measure 24 hour bio metric markers.

Markers like:

1. Steps in a Day
2. Calories in a Day
3. Links to Food Diaries and detailed Macro Nutrient profiles
4. All Day Stress and HRV
5. All Day Heart Rate
6. Floors Climbed

As technology improves the accuracy of Optical Heart Rate information will get better and better. We will soon be able to take a glance and see body temperature, respiration rate, oxygen consumption, blood glucose, fat utilization and blood lactate among other specific markers of health and performance. Our point here is that this DATA will be USELESS if we do not know what it means and how it affects us at the simplest level.

It all sounds like rocket science to most, but it is NOT. It is simple: we must reduce oxidation and inflammation by LEARNING how to manipulate the markers that raise and lower Oxidation and Inflammation. As we better gauge this we can reduce and eliminate the negative cascade of metabolic events and replace them with positive cascade of metabolic events. It all starts with USING TECHNOLOGY to our benefit to help guide and Master Our Lifestyle. It all STARTS with awareness and LEARNING!!

Power 2 Learn

My old saying to self is:

"We simply- do not know- what we <u>DO NOT</u> know, but we can LEARN"!

Experience is the best teacher, but wisdom is the ability to distinguish between what will work, and what will fail, what is a waste of time, and what is priceless.

Intelligence is the ability to discern, to make better choices. Success with the venture to **Master you Own Lifestyle** –Execute your Intelligence and **LEARN!**

Stop hitting your head on the wall and **LEARN**. Start measuring twice-and cutting once, start utilizing twice the thought, and half the effort to achieve four times the result. Learn about your metabolism and master some of the things we point out in this book and will constantly be updating as information changes at our website www.metafit.life and by Podcast at **"Power 2 Learn"** on iTunes or Google play, both are 100% FREE. Expand your awareness of opportunity to employ ever changing methodology toward metabolic fitness for life.

You are your own **Center of Mass** in your own four points of stability, literally and figuratively speaking. In Bio Mechanics we teach people how to be better aware of how and where you place your center of mass (COM) among four points of contact with the earth standing still.

Please try this right NOW!

I want you to stand up, keep reading, and stand up. I want you to be bare footed. I want you to stand with your feet shoulders width apart and I want you to number these four points that carry your **Center Of Mass** around each and every day of your life.

These four points are:

1. The rear part of your right foot #1
2. The front part of your right foot #2

3. The rear part of your left foot #3
4. The front part of your left foot #4

I want you to become better aware of your center of mass, and how your body positions itself among these **4-Points** right heel, right ball of foot, left heal, left ball of foot.

I want you to sway your body or **CENTER of MASS** among these 4 points in order from 1-4 and **SWAY** like a tall building in the wind.

- Sway back and right to position 1
- Sway right and front to position 2
- Sway left and rear to position 3
- Sway left and front to position 4
- Keep swaying around these four points to get your own personal feeling of balance within these points that support you standing and as you walk and run.

Your objective is to **FEEL** your mass shift as you transfer weight to these 4 points of stress that hold you up in life. Do it with your eyes closed and FEEL movement of mass among the points of contact you have with earth.

- Become better aware of self
- Better aware of balance and
- Much better Kinesthetic Awareness of movement.

Become better at sensing when you are **OFF** balance and in danger of over stressing any one point of support, both to standing and in Life whilst running, sprinting or walking.

Make sure you learn to distribute the stress, and support what is being called upon to- **HOLD** you up, and put you into a position to move swifter, jump higher and be stronger. Learn the **TRUE MEANING of BALANCE**.

Today is the first day of the rest of your life and you call the shots- for the most part. It is not always **WHAT** you do as much as it is **HOW YOU DO IT**.

Make good use of your time and technology. Don't waste your time with foolish programs and eating out of mail boxes, or rolling a tire around a room. Learn what is killing us and what will change the outcome. Improve your Bio Markers and DO it RIGHT the first time!

Make the right choice to:

- Oxidize the Fat
- Become Fat adapted
- Lower inflammation and oxidation a

With these changes you will reduce and even eliminate a cascade of nasty chronic conditions that bring chronic disease.

Improve your health- even improve your fitness, but **NOT** at the expense of your **HEALTH** as so many do (xfitters are you listening?)

LEARN and **TEACH**, teach what you learn- that you can support with evidence- show others how it works and do IT, be the example!

In closing

Use your head- before you abuse your body. A journey of 1,000 miles does start with a single step; just make sure you are pointing yourself in the right direction before you begin.

Life is precious, grab it and use the **Power 2 Learn**, contribute- and bathe yourself in knowledge with a humble heart, as you share what you learn, and what you do with the world around you.

Remember it is not always about the people, places and things around you, the food the situations of stress; it is your REACTION to them that matters. Physically your metabolic reaction and psychologically your emotional reaction.

Learn how your metabolism responds to physical activity, exercise, food and stress and learn to manipulate your lifestyle to redirect negatives into positives. Minus into plus and you will **WIN the Battle and win the War**!

When you find success, and I know you will, it is critical that you become the messenger we all need to be and **SHARE** what you learn. It all starts with the many little components you can choose to make part of your 16 hour life to:

Section #4 Summary:

I just got off the phone with my 87 year old mother and she does not want to live anymore! It breaks my heart that she has come to a place where she is so anxious, and depressed at the same time.

Each day brings her more misery of shortness of breath, panic and sadness. If there was ever a place to execute our intelligence and utilize a few tools of stress management it is **NOW!**

What are you equipping yourself with to identify and release yourself of health killing- acute and chronic stress?

How we deal with stress is critical. Sometimes it is a walk that relieves the emotional pain of stress. Sometimes it is a Hot Bath, or Yoga, or a long FFA Bike Ride, or a Race on Zwift or a session at M360.

It ALL counts! The 30,000ft Global View of your Lifestyle is what identifies you- as YOU! **Who are YOU?**

My point is we must be able to identify acute and chronic **STRESSORS** in **OUR** life and channel them accordingly.

Left un-checked stress will bring more and more inflammation/ oxidative stress and with it the cascade of cellular events that will not only destroy our body, but strip us of our mind and will to live; a very SAD and lonely place to be.

We can be better; we can alter outcomes with little things. Little things that become BIG things- we can choose to do each and every day like: effective relaxing deep breathing, dry brushing, walking and more.

Reach out and join us in a journey to **LEARN** with our book, our website blogs, and our podcast: **Power 2 Learn** on iTunes and Google play or on Podbean.

Let's do an interview and tell our listeners what **YOU** learned reading **THIS** book, more importantly what creative motivational wire did we stimulate for you to now **Teach** others a better way to live to improve-- rather than live to die.

We all need to get busy living! Let's make it count. God Bless!

Master your Lifestyle
And be
Metabolically Fit for Life!

Contact us at:
719.289.0351
tim@metafit.life
www.metafit.life
Power 2 Learn on:
Podbean, iTunes, and Google Play